handbook of child and adolescent psychiatric emergencies

by   **GORDON K. FARLEY, M.D.**
Associate Professor of Child Psychiatry
Director, Day Care Center, Division of Child Psychiatry
University of Colorado Medical Center
Denver, Colorado

LLOYD O. ECKHARDT, M.D.
Assistant Professor of Child Psychiatry and Pediatrics
Director, Pediatric Child Psychiatry and Psychology
Liaison Section, Division of Child Psychiatry
University of Colorado Medical Center
Denver, Colorado

FREDERICK B. HEBERT, M.D.
Assistant Clinical Professor of Child Psychiatry
Division of Child Psychiatry
University of Colorado Medical Center;
Director, Child and Adolescent Psychiatric Hospital Services
Denver General Hospital
Denver, Colorado

Medical Examination Publishing Co., Inc.
an Excerpta Medica company

969 Stewart Avenue   •   Garden City, New York 11530

Copyright © 1979 by
MEDICAL EXAMINATION
PUBLISHING CO. , INC.
an Excerpta Medica company

Library of Congress Card Number
79-88047

ISBN 0-87488-656-2

September, 1979

Printed in the United States of America

SIMULTANEOUSLY PUBLISHED IN:

Europe	:	HANS HUBER PUBLISHERS Bern, Switzerland
Japan	:	IGAKU-SHOIN Ltd. Tokyo, Japan
South and East Asia	:	TOPPAN COMPANY (S) Pte. Ltd. Singapore
United Kingdom	:	HENRY KIMPTON PUBLISHERS London, England

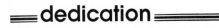

dedication

To Katharine, Susan, and Kathleen

═acknowledgments═

The authors wish to thank Carol Lee, Helen Wong, Aletha Arkie, Corrine Copeland, and Joy Maddox for their untiring typing and editorial efforts. We wish to thank the following people for reading portions of the manuscript and offering helpful comments: Dr. Dane G. Prugh, Dr. Stephen Dilts, Dr. Jerry M. Wiener, and Dr. Harry Umlauf. We also wish to thank Dr. Henry P. Coppolillo, Director, Division of Child Psychiatry, University of Colorado Medical Center, and Dr. Edmund G. Casper, Chairman, Department of Psychiatry, Denver General Hospital for their support and encouragement.

══with a contribution from══

══ with a contribution from ══

STEPHEN H. MEITUS, M.D.
Private Practice of Adult and Child Psychiatry
Clinical Instructor of Child Psychiatry
Division of Child Psychiatry
University of Colorado Medical Center
Denver, Colorado

══contents══════════════════════

CHAPTER I

INTRODUCTION

A child psychiatric emergency can be considered as a dangerous opportunity. This book is written to provide some guide-
lines for physicians and mental health workers who face this
difficult situation where possibilities exist for influencing a
family at a pivotal point. Such intervention can have a favorable or unfavorable effect on a family. The field of child psychiatric diagnosis and classification is currently in flux, and
there is much dissatisfaction regarding available classification
systems. In this book, a phenomenological or descriptive approach will be used to identify, describe and treat various child
psychiatric syndromes.

The book is divided into chapters on the following:

1. General principles of evaluation of child psychiatric emergencies
2. Reasons for referral to the emergency room
3. Child and adolescent psychiatric syndromes
4. Child and adolescent psychopharmacology

In general, each syndrome is discussed in the following manner:

1. General comments and/or a definition of the syndrome
2. Findings during the examination of the child and the parents
3. Differential diagnosis
4. Immediate treatment
5. Follow-up treatment

The various syndromes are arranged in alphabetical order for
easy reference. Bibliographies for all chapters appear together
at the end of the book, and are by chapter titles and by subhead-
ings as well, for Chapter IV.

Children's psychiatric emergencies are anxiety-provoking for
both the family and the emergency room worker. It is hoped
that the suggestions for treatment offered in this text may help

1

reduce some of that anxiety and lead to a therapeutic intervention. Some children and families can be helped significantly in
one emergency room visit. For many others, however, the
primary purpose of the emergency room visit is to help moti-
vate and assist the child and family in seeking and utilizing definitive and long-term treatment while they manage the immediate crisis.

A family that arrives in the emergency room seeking psychiatric help can be considered a family in a crisis. Usually, old
and familiar ways of handling stresses of everyday life have
become ineffective; and the family homeostasis or equilibrium
has become disturbed. In the crisis, the possibility exists that
the family may reconstitute or reorganize at a higher and more
effective level of development and coping. It is hoped that the
suggestions offered in this book will aid in this effort.

CHAPTER II

GENERAL PRINCIPLES OF
EMERGENCY ROOM EVALUATION

ATTITUDES OF PARENTS AND CHILDREN SEEKING HELP IN THE EMERGENCY ROOM:

Many parents and children who come to the emergency room for child psychiatric emergencies have sought help in a number of other settings without success or satisfaction. They are often frightened and angry and have exhausted most of their adaptive capacities. Their usual ways of handling family crises and problems have been found ineffective and are likely to have been abandoned. Since these old defenses and coping mechanisms previously used have not been replaced with new ones, the family may be unusually flexible and willing to try new ways of relating, disciplining, solving problems and adapting to stress.

STANCE AND ATTITUDE OF THE EXAMINER:

During the interview with the parents and the child, the interviewer should attempt to convey an attitude of serious concern; empathy with the difficulties the family is experiencing; confidence that something can be done about the difficulties and that things can be changed; and neutrality, regarding fault-finding within the family.

The focus in the emergency room can profitably be an attempt to define the specific problem that brings the family and child there. Often both parents and child may be vague in their complaints, and it is therefore helpful to refocus on what it is in the behavior of the child, or what it is in the psychological makeup of the child that bothers, disturbs or annoys them. Exploring and understanding the reasons for coming to this particular emergency room, at this particular time, can also be revealing and helpful.

The emergency room worker should be particularly sensitive to racial and ethnic differences and issues in parents and children coming for help. Several studies have demonstrated that black parents and black children tend to receive less than optimal treatment in mental health settings (Jackson, et al.) 1974; Warren, et al. , 1973; Gross and Herbert, 1969).

THE PSYCHIATRIC EXAMINATION:

The psychiatric examination conducted in the emergency room is a modification of the usual child and parent psychiatric examination. At times the interviewer may elect to see the entire family as a unit and include all of the family members who arrive at the emergency room. This procedure seems indicated when the presenting problem appears to be principally an interactional one between family members, such as a runaway, repeated suicide attempts, physical fighting within the family, etc. At other times it is important to see parents first, without the child, to obtain a present illness before interviewing the child. It may also be important to see the child first when the examiner anticipates that the child is suspicious, defensive and feels that the examiner is an agent of parents or other authority figures. In order to prevent precipitous departure, a highly agitated child should not be left alone at any time.

The following is a suggested outline for taking the present illness in an interview with the parents without the child being present. The information will not necessarily be collected in the order presented nor will all the information on the outline usually be collected, but the outline includes most areas of importance. (Adapted from Prugh, 1963.)

EXAMINATION OF THE PARENTS:

1. Decision to seek emergency care or referral (any circumstances pertaining to or connected with the referral or decision):

    a) Source of referral
    b) Factors precipitating referral or decision to seek care
    c) Previous treatment, if any, of parents and child
    d) Reactions of parents, overt or covert, to seeking help in the emergency room
    e) Reasons for choosing this emergency room

2. Description of mother and father:

    a) Physical description, appearance and grooming
    b) Predominant facial expressions or mannerisms
    c) Predominant patterns of interaction with interviewer and

with each other in the interview

3. Problems as presented by parents:
   a) Detailed description of the onset of the problem
   b) How parents attempted to handle the problem and the results of each attempt
   c) Their ideas of sources and reasons for the problems
   d) Their ideas as to the child's attitudes about his/her difficulties
   e) A specific and concrete description of the child's behavior including his/her behavior:
      (1) With each of them individually
      (2) With siblings
      (3) With peers
      (4) At school

4. Observations regarding the child:
   a) His disposition and temperament
   b) His interests and assets

5. Present and past family situation:
   a) Present: Family members, cultural orientation, economics. Recent events and changes influencing the family, such as divorce, death, separations, illnesses, moves, changes in employment situation, birth of a baby, anticipated loss etc. Reactions of parents and children to these events
   b) Past: Events and developments surrounding the child in infancy and childhood, especially any events similar to the precipitating events

6. Developmental history:
   a) Pregnancy and birth, planned or unplanned
   b) Illnesses and accidents
   c) Toilet training - when begun and how handled, outcome
   d) Weaning, feeding and sleeping
   e) Developmental landmarks, such as sitting alone, standing, walking, first words, first phrases, first sentences
   f) Unusual behaviors and age of onset of behaviors such as thumb sucking, rocking, feeding problems, colic, diarrhea, excessive crying, nightmares, masturbatory activity, speech difficulties, hyperactivity. How handled

7. School adjustment:
   a) Parents' complaints or observations
   b) Teachers' observations as obtained from parents
   c) Observations from the teachers, if needed

8. Diagnostic impressions:
   a) Impressions regarding parents as revealed in the interview
   b) View of the nature of the family interaction
   c) Impression of the family members' individual contributions to the clinical picture seen in the child
   d) Contributions from organic factors, such as mental retardation, brain damage, minimal brain dysfunction, drug toxicity, etc.
   e) Special strengths noted in the family
   f) Impressions regarding psychological mindedness, treatability and prognosis

EXAMINATION OF THE CHILD

Usually before the emergency room psychiatrist interviews the child, he/she has talked with the parents and has gained some information about the principal problems or complaints. Some beginning or tentative hypotheses regarding the origin and continuation of the problem have been formulated, and the interview with the child can be seen as an opportunity to confirm or refute these tentative hypotheses. Upon entering the emergency room, both the child and the parents will be frightened and confused. The examiner should maintain a stance of warmth, empathy and concern without participating in the helpless anxiety that the family experiences. Above all, the examiner should present a problem-solving orientation which demonstrates confidence that something can be done about the emergency the family is experiencing.

During the interview with the child, the examiner should be friendly and warm without being effusive, overwhelming or intrusive to a frightening extent. Questions and play (if the child is a younger child) should be age appropriate. Both direct questions and free play, as well as structured play, may be used where indicated. A suggested outline for recording the interview with the child follows:

1. Descriptions:
   a) Physical appearance of the child
   b) Interaction of the child with his/her parents observed:
      (1) In the waiting room
      (2) Separated from parents
      (3) Returned to parents
   c) Interaction with interviewer and the interview situation:
      (1) Initially
      (2) Later

       (3) Child's concept of why he/she is there
- d) Overt physiological manifestations of emotions
- e) Therapist's emotional response to the child

2. Behavioral description (from play, verbalization and direct observation):
   a) Affective tone
   b) Type of reaction (motor, speech, coordination)

3. Child's expressions about significant family relationships

4. Current adjustment as told by the child:
   a) Relationships to peers, teachers and other adults
   b) School, academic and social interests and dislikes
   c) Play activities, hobbies, sports and interests
   d) Identifications:
      (1) Whom he/she likes
      (2) What he/she wants to be, ambitions
      (3) What he/she thinks he/she is like

5. Fantasy expressions:
   a) Dreams
   b) Early memories
   c) Pets wished for and why
   d) Fables (Despert, 1937).
   e) Favorite TV programs or favorite movies
   f) Favorite stories, nursery rhymes, fairy tales
   g) Animal identification (what animal would you like to be and why?)

6. Clinical judgements:
   a) Physical deficits of psychological importance
   b) Drives: manifestations and intensity:
      (1) Aggression
      (2) Sexuality
   c) Anxiety
   d) Guilt, shame
   e) Ego functions:
      (1) Intelligence
      (2) Appropriateness of behavior to age level
      (3) Impulse control
      (4) Capacity to form a relationship
      (5) Ability to do reality testing
      (6) Defenses: against what, what types, age appropriateness
      (7) Awareness of feelings:
         (a) verbal acknowledgement

   (b)   communication through play

7. Revised clinical impressions of the child and family

8. Further diagnostic procedures needed

RESULTS OF FINDINGS, INTERPRETATION OF FINDINGS TO PARENTS AND RECOMMENDATIONS FOR TREATMENT:

Following the interview with the child (if the child is seen separately and following the parents), the interviewer should meet with the parents to discuss findings and recommendations. During this meeting, the interviewer should offer the parents a working hypothesis as to the origin, development, continuation and present status of the problem for which they are seeking help. This should be phrased in language free from psychiatric jargon and complicated medical terminology and suitable to the parents' educational and psychological level of understanding. Often asking parents to retell the interviewer what they understand of what he has told them offers an opportunity to assess the effectiveness of the interviewer's communication with them. Usually a good deal of work needs to be done before parents can begin to see themselves as a part of the problem for which they are seeking help. The emergency room worker should be especially careful to respect parental defenses. If definitive treatment is not offered in the emergency room further treatment should be recommended. The various treatment options, the amount of involvement expected of the family, and the setting in which the treatment will take place all need to be discussed with the family. If referral to a mental health center, outpatient clinic, private mental health practitioner or any other facility is made, it is necessary to make a telephone call at the time of referral and a later follow-up telephone call to assure completion of the referral.

CHAPTER III

PSYCHIATRIC EMERGENCIES IN CHILDHOOD

DEFINITION:

Mattsson and his co-workers (1969) define a child psychiatric emergency as a condition of sufficient emotional distress in a child which he/she, his/her family, or the referral source feel incapable of handling for even a few hours. Parental absence, anxiety or helplessness in the face of the stressful environmental condition provoke a situation which is experienced by the child as desertion and isolation. Other authors (Burks and Hoekstra, 1964) have found that children who have attempted suicide, those developing a psychosis, and those with an acute school phobia present bona fide emergency situations requiring prompt clinical intervention. The present authors agree that such situations are true emergencies and have added a number of other conditions and situations that may cause enough emotional distress to warrant prompt intervention.

GENERAL CHARACTERISTICS:

1. Childhood psychiatric emergencies may occur in the infancy period and then are often related to child abuse or neglect.

2. The peak incidence of childhood psychiatric emergencies occurs during the adolescent period of 12 to 18 years.

3. Mattsson and his co-workers (1969) emphasize the following characteristics:

   a) Girls are seen for psychiatric emergencies more commonly than boys: 60% vs 40%. This is due to the fact that girls account for a significantly higher percentage than boys of the reported psychiatric emergencies during the adolescent period. Of the preadolescent childhood psychiatric emergencies, boys slightly outnumber girls.

   b) The rate of family and self-referrals among child psychiatric emergencies seems to be 45%. In the adolescent group, self-referrals almost equal those made by physi-

9

cians, schools and other agencies.

c) Eighty percent of the patients are seen during weekdays and 20% during weekends.

d) No significant seasonal variation is observed.

e) Approximately 28% of the consultations take place between 8:00 P. M. and 8:00 A. M. , and these are usually for suicidal or psychotic adolescent patients.

f) The most common event leading to an emergency referral is an acute conflict between the child and his parental figures. Exacerbation of chronic physical illness or physical injury, including surgery, is the second most common precipitating factor. Other events triggering referral include school problems; sexual conflicts related to masturbation, menstruation, or homosexual contacts; conflicts with loss of heterosexual love objects; pregnancy; grief reactions; intoxication; and sexual molestation. Many of these problems reflect long-standing individual and family psychopathology (Morrison, 1969; Morrison and Collier, 1969).

PREDOMINANT PRECIPITATING SYMPTOMS
(Mattsson, et al. , 1969):

1. Suicidal behavior - 44%
2. Assaultive and destructive behavior - 19%
3. Marked anxiety and fears - 13%
4. Actions considered bizarre and confused - 10%
5. School refusal - 7%
6. Truancy or runaway - 7%

Slightly more than half of the emergencies (62%) are referred because of changes in mood and behavior, such as depression often associated with suicidal behavior, somatic complaints and fears. These children generally maintain satisfactory control of impulsive behavior toward the environment. The remaining referrals (38%) present with behavioral manifestations that are outwardly directed in an impulsive, often unmanageable fashion which indicates emotional conflicts acted out in an assaultive, delinquent, or truant manner. Children in the latter group, also at times, make suicidal attempts.

MAJOR DIAGNOSTIC CATEGORIES (Mattsson, et al. , 1969):

1. Adjustment reaction - 45%
2. Neurotic reactions - 27%

3. Personality disorders - 16%
4. Psychosis (all of the schizophrenic type) - 9%
5. Organic brain syndrome - 3%

FOLLOW-UP
(Mattsson, et al. , 1969):

Of the patients referred for evaluation of a psychiatric emergency, 33% were recommended for admission to inpatient facilities; 24% were referred to the child psychiatric OPD clinic;
23% to a social agency; 14% to return to the emergency room
p. r. n. ; and 6% to the court.

CHAPTER IV

SPECIFIC CHILD PSYCHIATRIC EMERGENCIES

ACUTE DRUG ABUSE

GENERAL COMMENTS:

1. In recent years there has been a widespread increase in acute drug abuse (Beebe, 1975). Acute drug abuse has been defined as the use of drugs to produce altered states of consciousness which lead to social, emotional or legal problems.

2. Alcohol still remains the most widely abused drug; however, marijuana use has increased dramatically to a stable level, and it is now second only to alcohol in frequency of abuse. In one report of drivers arrested in California for erratic driving, one-fourth of the drivers were found to have the active ingredient of marijuana (tetrahydrocannabinol) in their blood (Cohen, 1977).

3. The demand by youth for drugs in order to "turn on" has resulted in the use of many drugs including alcohol, other sedative hypnotics, hallucinogens, various types of stimulants and organic solvents.

   a) The sedative hypnotics include barbiturates (yellows, reds, rainbows) and barbiturate-like drugs, such as methaqualone (soapers).

   b) The hallucinogens include lysergic acid diethylamide (LSD, acid) mescaline (peyote, cactus), psilocybin (magic mushroom) and phencyclidine (PCP, angel dust).

   c) Marijuana (pot, grass, hash) seems to act as both a sedative hypnotic and a mild hallucinogen. It commonly produces euphoria and some sedation as well as "illusions," but it rarely produces true hallucinations.

d) Dimethyltryptamine (DMT) and 2,5-dimethoxy-4-methyl-amphetamine (DOM or STP for serenity, tranquility and peace) are chemically related to the amphetamines but generally produce a clinical picture more like the hallucinogens. They are less potent than LSD but more potent than mescaline.

e) Stimulants include amphetamines (speed, dexedrine, white crosses), methylphenidate (Ritalin), a host of anorectic drugs (Pre-Sate, Tenuate) and cocaine (coke, snow).

f) Volatile substances include aerosal sprays (paint, hair, cooking oil), cryogenic chilling fluids (Freon), solvents (gasoline, paint thinner, lighter fluid) and toluene (airplane glue, plastic and rubber cement).

g) Narcotic analgesics include morphine (morf, Miss Emma) and heroin (smack, stuff, junk).

h) Anticholinergic drugs include atropine and scopolamine (scope) available in a myriad of over-the-counter cold and sleep preparations.

HISTORY:

1. Since many of these drugs are manufactured illegally or illegally purchased, an adequate history is often impossible to obtain either from the user or his/her cohorts, as legal reprisals are feared.

2. Certain drugs such as alcohol and marijuana are likely to be used in the context of a social interaction.

3. Younger users are likely to use the more available drugs such as anticholinergic agents, marijuana, sedative hypnotics or other drugs they can find around the house.

4. Older or more experienced users or those with more money to spend often use powerful synthetic stimulants: cocaine or heroin.

5. A history of legal problems increases the likelihood of amphetamine or narcotic use.

6. Historically, the progression of drug abuse has depended heavily on street availability. This progression has gone from alcohol to acid to speed to, to heroin to co-

caine to alcohol.

7. Currently, PCP (phencyclidine) is in widespread use.

8. Adulteration of drugs increases profits, and therefore, the average acute drug abuser will have mixed symptoms based on contamination of the active ingredients with sugar, lactose, strychnine, talc, camphor, or most commonly, some anticholinergic agent.

9. Laboratory tests are primarily available for the diagnosis of alcohol, sedative hypnotic and narcotic analgesic abuse.

DIFFERENTIAL DIAGNOSIS:

1. Acute alcohol or sedative hypnotic intoxication alone or in combination with other substances must always be considered because of the wide availability of these drugs. The symptoms vary with the amount ingested, the mode of administration, and the rate at which the substance is metabolized. Because it is quickly metabolized, alcohol should be suspected when a fairly rapid progression of changes in mental status is seen over a period of observation. This may occur even though the characteristic breath odor of alcohol intoxication is absent. In equivocal cases, laboratory confirmation is easily obtained; however, the level of intoxication correlates only grossly with the degrees of behavioral change. The patient with a mild degree of intoxication is usually friendly and chatty. At higher levels, he may be fearful or withdrawn and finally at very high levels, stuporous or comatose. The motor effects are first manifested by mild dysarthria, progressing to slurred speech, general lethargy and finally respiratory depression. Affect progresses from euphoria and flight of ideas through insecurity to depression. Cognitive impairment begins with difficulty in making fine social discriminations and progresses to an inability to answer simple questions and complete disorientation.

These patients need to be differentiated from those who are in acute withdrawal from alcohol or sedative hypnotics. One can differentiate withdrawal from intoxication if one remembers that rebound CNS oversensitivity will be seen in withdrawal, whereas CNS depression will be seen in intoxication. Individuals who are withdrawing will often take some sedative hypnotic in an effort to forestall withdrawal. Therefore, one may have to wait for some progression of symptoms be-

fore making a definitive diagnosis. The progression of
symptoms again depends on the agent. Withdrawal symptoms may start within a few hours after reducing or discon-
tinuing the ingestion of alcohol but always begin within
72 hours. Barbiturate symptoms usually appear within two
or three days, while symptoms resulting from withdrawal
of benzodiazepines commonly take several days, but may
take up to two weeks to appear. The rebound CNS sensitiv-
ity results in many physical symptoms beginning with complaints of weakness and nausea. The patient is noted to be
restless and tremulous or in severe cases to have an actual
seizure. Medical examination reveals an increase in temperature and pulse rate, and these findings are the best
guide to an impending delirium (Thomas and Freedman,
1964; Victor, 1968). If the pulse is over 120 and the temperature over 100°F or if the patient is in poor physical
condition, medical consultation is imperative. Untreated
severe alcohol or sedative hypnotic withdrawal can be fatal,
and treatment must always be carried out in a hospital. Patients in withdrawal have an anxious and irritable affect, and
their sleep is disturbed. Cognitively, they may have perceptual disturbances from tinnitus (most common) to click-
ing sounds. In more serious cases there may be hallucinations of a voice which speaks in the third person ("What's
he up to?") in contrast to hallucinations in the first or second
person as seen in schizophrenia. Auditory hallucinations are
usually followed later by disorientation and still later by other
signs of withdrawal, including visual and tactile hallucinations.

2. In marijuana intoxication, consistent physical findings are
an increase in heart rate, a dilation of conjunctival blood
vessels and normal-sized pupils. Initial restlessness is replaced by detachment, so that observation should include a
careful mental status examination in order to reveal the extensive cognitive changes. At low doses, there are illusions
of all five senses: sight, sound, smell, taste and touch. At
higher doses, rapidly shifting illusionary images, fragmen-
tary thoughts and a sense of increased insight, despite memory impairment (temporary amnesia), occur. At very high
doses, there is an intensification of the cognitive disturbances so that the usual affect state of dreamy, carefree
relaxation is replaced by rapidly changing emotions and
frank hallucinations.

3. LSD or mescaline intoxication is usually characterized by
cognitive changes with visual illusions of changing colors
and shapes. With larger ingestions, frank hallucinations

occur. With pure LSD or mescaline, physical effects are mild anticholinergic responses with dilated pupils and a transient or mild increase in pulse rate and blood pressure. Dry palms and tactile hallucinations are not seen unless the hallucinogen has been contaminated with an anticholinergic drug. There is usually increased motor activity in response to the illusions. The prominent affect is marked anxiety in response to awe, dread, horror or loathing which seem to be directly induced by the drug.

4. In phencyclidine intoxication (PCP), specific physical signs are many and are seen more often than with other intoxications (Showalter and Thornton, 1977). Pupils are usually of normal size, but occasionally, they may show a constriction that is commonly associated with nystagmus and ptosis. Slurred speech, ataxia, partial analgesias and paresthesias are common when small amounts are ingested. With increasing doses there is peripheral muscle weakness progressing to muscular rigidity or catatonic posturing, and at toxic levels, progression to myoclonus, convulsions and coma. Blood pressure is increased. Respirations are stimulated at low doses but depressed at higher doses. Sensory impairment precedes the psychological effects. The first psychological symptoms are cognitive with changes in body image. Patients frequently describe sensations of total body contraction and elongation or feelings that the limbs are floating away. Later, disorganization with thought blocking, impairment of proverb interpretation and serial subtraction occurs. This finding is in contrast to LSD intoxication which produces hallucinations but no primary thought disturbance. Cognitive effects may not appear for several days, and anterograde amnesia is frequently seen on follow-up. The initial affect seen with large or small doses is euphoria. Later and most commonly with large doses, the effect is anxiety. Still later, depersonalization, feelings of isolation and depression occur and persist for hours. At even higher doses, hostility and negativism progress to apathy or catatonia. The slow onset and slow decline of behavioral toxicity associated with the above physical manifestations should raise suspicion of PCP ingestion.

5. Stimulant intoxication produces the physical signs of an increase in heart rate, blood pressure, deep tendon reflexes and sweating, as well as dilated but reactive pupils. The patient's affect varies from anxiety at low doses to irritability or combativeness at higher levels. Cognitively, the patient's thought processes are accelerated, and there may

be pressure of speech or even mild confusion. Disorientation or auditory hallucinations in the form of acute paranoid psychosis are seen only in more serious intoxications. If the patient is acutely psychotic with hallucinations but oriented, only laboratory exam and/or a period of hospitalization may allow one to distinguish stimulant intoxication from paranoid schizophrenia.

6. Acute solvent intoxication commonly produces the physical sensations of blurred vision and a ringing or buzzing in the ears. Reverberations or echoing of internal noises such as swallowing or breathing may also be present. If, in addition to the above, there is swelling of the nasal or oral mucous membranes, toluene intoxication is likely. The patient's affect is usually giddy, although with more severe intoxication, stupor or coma may result. Chronic users may present with seizures and show laboratory evidence or physical signs of liver disease, anemia or bone marrow depression. Cognitively, most acute and chronic cases will be disoriented to place, as well as time.

7. Adolescents intoxicated with narcotic analgesics tend to be older than the users of other drugs. The physical signs include nausea, lethargy and drowsiness at lower doses. With higher doses, one may see vomiting despite lethargy, somnolence, pinpoint pupils and respiratory depression. The lack of slurred speech and ataxia, even at the point of respiratory depression, helps distinguish this condition from sedative hypnotic intoxication. Affect ranges from euphoria or mild dysphoria at low doses, to dreamy withdrawal and contentment at high doses. Euphoria in the presence of vomiting is referred to as the "good sick" among addicts. Cognitively, the impairment is mild, as compared to that of other intoxications; the addicts show only a lack of motivation and an inability to concentrate on mental tasks. Seldom, if ever, is there actual disorientation. Massive overdoses present with coma, pinpoint pupils and severe respiratory depression, and call for emergency medical management.

Narcotic withdrawal presents with many physical signs, most of which are explained by rebound cholinergic activity. Runny nose, tearing eyes with dilated pupils, profuse sweating, crampy diarrhea, and nausea without vomiting, are prominant. Later, gooseflesh ("cold turkey"), restlessness and tremor appear. The signs just mentioned are known collectively as "nonpurposive behavior." This is accompanied by an affect of acute anxiety and irritability and a cognitive

state in which the patient's hypervigilance and insomnia direct him toward obtaining more of the drug. The resulting
marked exaggeration of the physical symptoms is known as
"purposive behavior."

8. Anticholinergic intoxication displays several physical signs
as a direct result of the drug action. Heart rate and temperature are elevated, and pupils are widely dilated. Depending on the amount of drug used, the pupils react slightly
or not at all to light, in contrast to the dilated but reactive
pupils seen in pure hallucinogen intoxication. The patient
may continually request water because of dry mucosa, and
facial flushing may be prominent. Difficulty in urinating is
common, but bladder paralysis is seen only at high doses.
The lack of sweating is all the more striking in view of the
patient's affect, one of marked anxiety, usually secondary
to a florid delirium. Cognitively, the patients are often disoriented to place as well as time, and visual and tactile hallucinations are common. Auditory hallucinations are unusual; this fact helps differentiate anticholinergic toxicity
from alcohol withdrawal. The cognitive symptoms can be
cleared by an injection of physostigmine, but the serious
side-effects of this drug, for example, seizures (which can
also be seen in highly toxic doses of anticholinergics) miti-
gate against its routine use. An old poem aptly summarizes
the anticholinergic intoxication:

> Red as a beet
> Dry as a bone
> Mad as a hatter
> Hot as a stone

ACUTE TREATMENT:

1. General principles:

    a) Since all patients with an organic brain syndrome have
    disorientation as a prominent symptom, one of the most
    important parts of treatment is to help them reorient
    themselves.

        (1) The patient should be seen in a part of the emergen-
        cy room that is quiet, out of the mainstream of ac-
        tivity, and well lighted.

        (2) The clinician should introduce himself each time he
        sees the patient and reorient that patient to his/her

surroundings, including place and time.

(3) The clinician should try to get the patient to put his/ her experience into words to help the patient gain some control over his/her feelings and behavior. (Phencyclidine intoxication may be an exception (see pp. 22-23).

(4) If possible, friends or relatives of the patient (who themselves are not acutely intoxicated or agitated) should be allowed to stay with the patient.

b) Most acutely intoxicated patients can be "talked down" if there is adequate time (four to eight hours).

c) Since many emergency rooms are pressed for space, some patients may need to be hospitalized or medicated to decrease the anxiety associated with their intoxication. Any child or adolescent who has been medicated should be released only to the custody of a competent adult who can observe and be responsible for him/her during the 24 hours after discharge.

2. Acute alcohol intoxication is so common that it does not usu- ally attract medical attention by itself. There are no special symptoms seen in children or adolescents. On occasion, a youngster under peer group pressure may ingest a consid- erable quantity of high-proof distillates within a short space of time, and present unconscious in the emergency room with blood alcohol levels in excess of 400 mg%. Usually gas- tric irritation tends to limit the alcohol level by causing vomiting. It is not known whether the youth simply con- sciously tries to avoid vomiting or whether rapid absorp- tion leads to unconsciousness. An unconscious patient is a medical emergency that needs appropriate medical manage- ment. In cases short of unconsciousness, the patient must be frequently observed to be certain that he/she is not pro- gressing toward coma.

Alcohol withdrawal symptoms are not common in adoles- cents, probably because the syndrome seems to require that the individual drink considerable quantities for a lengthy pe- riod of time. Though adolescents may drink large amounts, they usually have not been drinking for a long enough period of time to generate an abstinence syndrome. If there are symptoms of withdrawal, such as tremulousness, fever or disorientation, detoxification is required. The following is a model adapted from Beebe (1975):

a) Thiamine, 100 mg, is given IM initially and then 50 mg three times a day orally, along with vitamin B complex daily.

b) The patient is put on a bland diet to reduce gastritis.

c) Aluminum hydroxide, 30 cc, can be given every four hours, as necessary, for gastric distress.

d) Fluids should be given in moderation for the first 24 hours because there is an overall retention of fluid. The excess extracellular fluid is lost in about four days in well-nourished patients.

e) Environmental support in the form of a general hospital or pediatric ward is necessary. An adolescent psychiatric ward with medical backup is ideal. Psychologically minded personnel are best able to treat the patient, because they see the patient as a person suffering from a psychiatric illness and do not pass moral judgment on him.

f) Psychopharmacological treatment is necessary to suppress withdrawal symptoms and provide a smooth withdrawal. Sedative hypnotics including paraldehyde, chloral hydrate and the benzodiazepines; chlordiazepoxide (Librium), and clorazepate (Tranxene) have been used. Sedating antihistamines, such as hydroxyzine (Vistaril), seem less effective (Dilts, 1977). Phenothiazines, such as Thorazine, have been shown to be inferior and should not be used (Kaim, et al. 1969). The benzodiazepines are currently preferred. Despite reports that they are erratically and incompletely absorbed IM, this has not been a problem in practice, probably because most patients can and should be given their medication orally. Librium, up to 200 mg/70 kg, can be given in the first 24-hour period in divided doses, such as 50 mg orally or IM every four to six hours. On the second day of withdrawal, Librium 25 mg/70 kg can be given orally every four to six hours as necessary, and this can be reduced to 25 mg/70 kg twice daily on the third day, and then discontinued if there is no further evidence of toxic withdrawal. Ninety percent of convulsions will occur in the first seven to forty-eight hours if they are related to withdrawal. Alcohol withdrawal symptoms resolve within four to five days if properly treated. Dilantin is not of value in protecting against withdrawal seizures.

g) Chronic, heavy alcohol intake in a pregnant adolescent may result in the fetal alcohol syndrome in the newborn child (Jones and Smith, 1973).

3. In acute intoxication with sedative hypnotics, the patient is observed over a period of time to be certain, from vital signs and mental status observations, that a lethal or dangerous amount has not been taken.

If addiction is suspected, the amount of drug used is not known, and there are no signs of intoxication, a test dose of 200 mg/70 kg of pentobarbital can be given IM. The patient is observed and his condition is noted over a 60-minute period of time. If the patient falls asleep, withdrawal from chronic use is unlikely. If the patient is awake but shows signs of intoxication, such as slurred speech or ataxia, he has probably been using less than 600 mg/day of pentobarbital or its equivalent. If he is comfortable and has normal speech and gait but shows minimal lateral nystagmus, about 800 mg/day have been used. If there is no response to the test dose, 1000 mg or more per day of pentobarbital have been used. If there is any evidence of addiction, the patient must be admitted to a special drug detoxification unit or general medical ward.

The amount of daily intake estimated from the test dose should be given in four to six divided doses of pentobarbital or its equivalent over 24 hours. The patient is observed during this period, and depending on whether the patient appears intoxicated or begins withdrawal signs, the dose is adjusted to get a better estimate of the patient's addictive level. Often this process takes over 24 hours, and it is best to keep the patient mildly intoxicated. After stabilization, the dose is decreased by 10% or 100 mg pentobarbital every one or two days. If any withdrawal symptoms appear, the dose is stabilized until withdrawal symptoms disappear and withdrawal is reinstituted at a slower pace. Often the entire process takes up to two weeks and should include medical management of fluid and electrolyte balance, as well as a safe environment and follow-up counseling to prevent the common return to sedative hypnotic abuse.

Other sedative hypnotics are withdrawn in a similar fashion. Benzodiazepines have a long half-life, as noted, and the late appearance of seizures may require a more gradual reduction of dose, the use of phenobarbital (32 mg) or the use of the specific benzodiazepine itself.

Table IV. 1, adapted from Smith and Wesson (1971) gives the oral hypnotic dose of a number of sedative hypnotics which can be used as an equivalent to 32 mg of phenobarbital. For example, if the patient reports taking ten 500 mg Doriden tablets per day, he/she would need ten 32 mg phenobarbital tablets per day, for stabilization. Divided into four doses, the starting withdrawal dose would be 64 mg at 6:00 A. M. , 12:00 noon and 6:00 P. M. , and 128 mg at 12:00 midnight. The midnight dose is always the largest and the last to be reduced, as the total dose is reduced by 32 mg phenobarbital per day. If the patient shows signs of phenobarbital toxicity (nystagmus, slurred speech, ataxia), his/her next dose should be omitted and the total dose cut in half.

TABLE IV. 1
Oral hypnotic dose equivalents to 32 mg phenobarbital

TRADE NAME	GENERIC NAME	ORAL HYPNOTIC DOSE IN MG
Seconal	Secobarbital	100
Nembutal	Pentobarbital	100
Noctec	Chloral hydrate	1000
Equanil, Miltown	Meprobamate	800
Doriden	Glutethimide	500
Librium, SK-Lygen	Chlordiazepoxide	75
Valium	Diazepam	15

4. Patients intoxicated with hallucinogens including marijuana, LSD and mescaline do not usually need any medication. If the patient is acutely agitated and a quiet, secure room is unavailable, Valium 5-10 mg IM/70 kg can be given. Thorazine was used formerly, but interactions between the Thorazine and contaminents in the hallucinogen sometimes led to untoward reactions, such as hypotension or shock.

5. With phencyclidine intoxication, at least some authors (Showalter and Thornton, 1977) have mentioned that toxicity appears to require some external input to create agitation. For mild intoxication, he recommends only observation with minimal stimulation, for one to two hours. Repeated attempts at "talking the patient down" may only increase anxiety, and the most successful method has been to place the patient in a quiet, dimly lit room. A letter from the National Institute

of Drug Abuse (DuPont, 1977) supports this method for behavioral control and also lists numerous problems associated with PCP overdose, including respiratory depression, seizures or status epilepticus, intracerebral hemorrhage, hypertensive encephalopathy, hyperpyrexia and cardiac arrest. Patients with these problems need to be managed on a medical or pediatric ward and some on an intensive care basis. If sedation is necessary, phenothiazines should be avoided because of significant blood pressure decreases. Valium, 5-10 mg IM/70 kg, can be used and is useful for myoclonus and seizures. If Valium is not effective, Haldol, 5-10 mg orally or IM/70 kg, can be used, since hypotension is not a problem with its use. Showalter (1977) notes that patients with pre-existing thought disorders are most likely to require Haldol.

6. Patients intoxicated with stimulants usually need only the general measures just outlined. Thorazine and Haldol are dopamine antagonists and thus specific for amphetamine-type drugs. Adulterants, however, make the use of Thorazine hazardous. Haldol, 5 mg/70 kg IM, can be given if the patient is psychotic.

7. There is no specific treatment for the acutely intoxicated solvent abuser, except that medications are to be avoided. If carbon tetrachloride was used, urinary output should be monitored (Cohen, 1975). In chronic users, anemia and liver damage are common and need medical evaluation.

8. Anticholinergic intoxication can produce a florid delirium with markedly abnormal behavior. The physician's temptation to use medication is strong, especially in the face of emergency room personnel who want to "do something about that noisy patient." In general, medication should be avoided, and if the patient is so agitated as to be a danger to himself or others, it may be best to admit him overnight. If sedation is necessary, Valium, 5-10 mg IM/70 kg, can be given. Paradoxical excitement from Valium is unusual but has been reported in young children. Medications with their own anticholinergic activity, such as Thorazine or sedating antihistamines, such as Vistaril or Benadryl, are contraindicated. Physostigmine salicylate (Antilirium) is a tertiary amine that crosses the blood-brain barrier and competes for receptor sites with the centrally-acting anticholinergic intoxicant. When given in adequate amounts, it clears the delirium, but its own cholinergic stimulation may result in hypersalivation, increased bronchial secretions,

dyspnea, abdominal colic and bradycardia. The most common effects are nausea and vomiting. If given too quickly intravenously, it can induce seizures. Relative contraindications include diabetes, gangrene, glaucoma, coronary artery disease, heart block, hypothyroidism, asthma or other respiratory diseases, peptic ulcer disease, ulcerative colitis, mechanical bowel or bladder obstruction and pregnancy. Some authors would make its use routine and even recommend giving peripherally-acting anticholinergics IM simultaneously to block the peripheral effects of physostigmine (Granacher and Baldessarini, 1975). It seems wiser to adopt a conservative approach and limit the use of physostigmine to cases of serious cardiac arrhythmias or repeated seizures. It can be given slowly IV (0.5-2.0 mg/70kg at a rate of no more than 1 mg/min), or given IM 0.5-2.0 mg/70 kg, and repeated in intervals from 30 minutes to 2 hours until the patient improves or shows signs of cholinergic toxicity. Overdoses of two psychiatric drugs, Mellaril and Elavil, are most likely to produce cardiac arrhythmias, in addition to anticholinergic toxic delirium.

9. Since narcotic intoxications usually involve impairment of vital functions, nearly all will involve medical or pediatric management. Children are more sensitive to respiratory depression than are young adults and may need artificial respiratory support. Narcan (naloxone hydrochloride), 0.01 mg/kg, is a narcotic antagonist that does not cause respiratory depression and can be given as a diagnostic test intravenously and repeated in three minutes. If the patient is unimproved after three doses, opiate toxicity is not the cause of the coma. Chronic abusers who have lost their tolerance to narcotics by being off them for a time, and small children who take their parents' supply of narcotics accidently, are at the greatest risk for severe intoxication or overdose.

The acute treatment of narcotic withdrawal involves symptomatic treatment of the physical signs of withdrawal, including diarrhea and abdominal cramping, with agents such as Pro-Banthine (propantheline bromide), 15-30 mg/70 kg, orally. A one- or two-day supply of Valium can be given for agitation or insomnia. Methadone should not be given, but a referral should be made to a methadone treatment program for evaluation for withdrawal or maintenance. Narcotic addiction in a pregnant adolescent may result in the fetal abstinence syndrome in a newborn infant.

FOLLOW-UP TREATMENT:

1. Follow-up treatment should include education and psychotherapy, where indicated, for concurrent emotional illness.

2. Residential treatment may be necessary for a chronic drug-abusing adolescent.

: :

ADOLESCENT SCHIZOPHRENIA

GENERAL COMMENTS
(Babgigian, 1975):

1. Schizophrenia continues to be a devastating, chronic and incapacitating disease.

2. Each year, between 100,000 and 200,000 Americans are afflicted with the disease.

3. Since the lifetime or overall prevalence is about 1%, approximately 2 million persons suffer from schizophrenia in the United States.

4. About 1 million persons require some psychiatric attention, and 60% of these require hospitalization in any given year.

5. Schizophrenia is most prevalent between the ages of 15 and 54.

6. Incidence and prevalence rates are higher for nonwhites.

7. The prevalence rates are highest among the lower socioeconomic classes.

8. The probability of developing schizophrenia is higher for relatives of schizophrenics than among the general population. The probability is 12% for children with one schizophrenic parent and 35-44% for children having two schizophrenic parents.

9. The incidence of schizophrenia has remained unchanged in the United States over the past 100 years.

HISTORY
(Weiner, 1975):

1. Retrospective studies of schizophrenic adults show that they have had several different developmental histories.

2. A typical history is that of a schizoid, premorbid personality. As a child, he/she is said to have been quiet and passive with few friends; as an adolescent, a daydreamer, introverted, and shut-in (schizoid group).

3. Another group may show a style of clinging to their mothers and possibly sharing their mothers' bedrooms until late adolescence. These children also had nightmares, were enuretic and became fearful when away from home (separation anxiety group).

4. Another group seemed asocial, shameless and lacking ordinary social propriety from an early age (asocial group).

5. The last group was overly compliant and concerned about the opinions of parents and peers. These children were also afraid to express themselves, overly mannered, and anxious to please (dependent group).

6. The common elements of the various groups seem to be a defect in relating to other people and a tendency to daydream.

7. Ordinarily, family members relate to each other according to assigned roles. In the family of the schizophrenic the number of these roles is limited, and family members may shift from one role to another within this limited framework. This type of relationship is known as pseudomutuality (Singer and Wynne, 1963).

8. At times the child may be made to feel helpless and enraged in a battle with one parent (usually the mother), while the other parent is also unable to help solve the problems. Or, there may be two conflicting communications from the same person. One is usually verbal, and the other nonverbal. The child feels he/she cannot win. This style of relating is known as the double bind (Bateson, et al. 1956).

EXAMINATION OF PARENTS (Lehmann, 1975):

1. Parents may report the following:

   a) The child was considered "especially good" because he/

she was always obedient and never in any mischief.

b) The child did well in grade school, and, at first, in junior and/or senior high school, but more recently grades have fallen off.

c) The patient has gradually become more withdrawn, preferring to spend time in his/her room.

d) The patient has had few dates, has not learned to dance and has few or no close friends of either sex.

e) The patient avoids all competitive sports but likes to go to the movies, or is an avid reader of books on philosophy or psychology.

2. Parents may also report that blood relatives suffered from schizophrenia or "dementia praecox," or the parents themselves may show signs of schizophrenia.

EXAMINATION OF THE ADOLESCENT
(Lehmann, 1975):

1. The adolescent may be agitated or quiet but always seems to be in his/her own world.

2. He/she may also seem confused, but if questioned, and willing to answer, is well oriented.

3. The adolescent may be experiencing hallucinations. Auditory hallucinations are frequently reported (over 30% of the time), and he/she may appear to be listening to voices. With younger adolescents, it is helpful to ask, "Are your eyes or ears playing tricks on you?" Visual hallucinations are reported between 4% and 10% of the time.

4. Difficulty in sleeping is frequently reported (over 30% of the time) and is commonly due to nightmares.

DIAGNOSIS AND DIFFERENTIAL PROGNOSIS:

1. Feighner and his co-workers (1972) devised diagnostic criteria for schizophrenia. Their criteria are as follows:

a) Both of the following are necessary:

(1) A chronic illness, with at least six months of symp-

toms prior to the index evaluation, without return to the premorbid level of psychosocial adjustment

(2) Absence of a period of depressive or manic symptoms, sufficient to qualify for affective disorder or probable affective disorder

b) The patient must have at least one of the following:

(1) Delusions or hallucinations without significant perplexity or disorientation associated with them

(2) Verbal production that makes communication difficult because of a lack of logical or understandable organization. (In the presence of muteness, the diagnostic decision must be deferred.)

c) At least three of the following manifestations must be present for a diagnosis of "definite" schizophrenia, and two for a diagnosis of "probable" schizophrenia:

(1) Single
(2) Poor premorbid social adjustment or work history
(3) Family history of schizophrenia
(4) Absence of alcoholism or drug abuse within one year of onset of psychosis
(5) Onset of illness prior to age 40

2. Schizophrenia must be differentiated from manic-depressive disorder, drug intoxications and withdrawal, and neurological (organic) disorders.

3. Manic-depressive illness commonly presents with euphoria, hyperactivity, pressured speech and distractibility, and presents no difficulty in differentiation from schizophrenia. Mania may, however, present with irritability, excitement and grandiosity of delusional proportions. About one quarter of all manic patients will present with delusions or hallucinations. With these presentations, it is tempting indeed to label the patient as schizophrenic. Persons relying on Bleulerian criteria of loose associations, impaired affect, ambivalence and autism are especially prone to make this error when dealing with manic adolescents (who, in general, are likely to present with an affect of irritability rather than euphoria) and particularly with those adolescents of a culture different from that of the examiner's. This occurs because examiners are more likely to label culture-different behavior as deviant and autistic and therefore, possibly schizophrenic.

4. Acute drug intoxications are sometimes confused with schizophrenia. LSD, drugs with central anticholinergic activity, and more recently, phencyclidine, can cause a psychosis but almost always do so with visual hallucinations, an accompanying disorientation to time, and impairment in recent memory (as demonstrated in serial subtractions) which are only rarely seen in schizophrenia. Phencyclidine and anticholinergic drugs often give rise to tactile hallucinations (formication), and phencyclidine also shows focal neurological signs, such as vertical nystagmus and ptosis.

5. Withdrawal of sedative hypnotics or alcohol on rare occasions leads to auditory hallucinations with a clear sensorium, but there are usually physical signs of withdrawal, such as elevated temperature and tremor which are absent in schizophrenia.

6. Psychotic behavior has been associated with trauma, infection, tumor, vascular disease, epilepsy and degenerative diseases. Except for psychotic behavior associated with epilepsy, memory deficit, confusion and fluctuating levels of consciousness should make differentiation from schizophrenia routine. Other neurological signs, such as tremor, myoclonic jerks and asterixis must be kept in mind. (Pincus and Tucker, 1978). Differentiation from epilepsy may be difficult if the patient's state makes it impossible to obtain a history of epilepsy, and there are no signs of seizure activity (Slater et al. 1963). An EEG may be obtained but is of only limited usefulness, since it may be normal in epileptic psychosis.

7. There are no definitive psychological tests for schizophrenia (Zubin, et al., 1965).

ACUTE TREATMENT:

1. Most adolescents undergoing a first acute schizophrenia reaction are best managed in a hospital setting. An adolescent psychiatric service with special facilities and staff can be helpful.

2. Some adolescents having their first psychotic episode, and many having a recurrence of their psychosis, can be managed on an outpatient basis if the following criteria are met:

   a) The environment is supportive, including family and school.

b) The physician is familiar with the patient and can closely monitor his treatment, including medications.

c) The patient does not manifest homicidal or suicidal ideation.

FOLLOW-UP TREATMENT:

1. Antipsychotic medications are necessary but not sufficient in the treatment of schizophrenia. Any antipsychotic medication may be used (see Chapter V, pp. 147-152 for details). The most common error in the use of medications is the use of an inadequate dose (Davis, 1976). Eventually, about 40% of schizophrenic patients should be able to be drug-free (Davis, 1975).

2. Milieu therapy can be helpful. However, an adolescent milieu with a majority of patients suffering from hyperkinetic or aggressive behavior disorders, an assertive staff, frequent group meetings, and assaultive music may be overwhelming for an isolated and withdrawn adolescent (Van Putten, 1973).

3. Some adolescent schizophrenic patients may benefit from individual psychotherapy with certain psychotherapists. However, the effectiveness of psychotherapy alone in the treatment of adolescent schizophrenia has not been demonstrated (May, 1976). It is important to remember that psychotherapy, like other forms of treatment, has its indications and contraindications.

4. Behavior therapy has been of value in some cases of schizophrenia but has not been adequately evaluated in controlled studies (May, 1976).

5. Vigorous outpatient aftercare programs such as vocational rehabilitation and halfway houses, in combination with antipsychotic medication, can be effective in maintaining patients in the community and preventing a downward spiral (May, 1976).

6. An underlying assumption in any effective treatment is the maintainence of a good therapeutic alliance with the adolescent patient and his family.

: :

ANOREXIA NERVOSA

GENERAL COMMENTS AND DEFINITION:

Anorexia nervosa is an obsessional preoccupation with the desire to be thin. The syndrome is observed most frequently during adolescence or early adulthood (Bruch, 1973). It may, however, have its onset during the late latency period. The conflict over eating becomes intensified and may be extremely resistant to treatment. The incidence of this syndrome has been reported to be 1.3 per 100,000 (Bliss, 1975).

HISTORY:

1. Anorexia nervosa occurs predominantly in girls but occasionally may be seen in boys.

2. There is often a history of early feeding problems.

3. The onset often occurs in relation to a strenuous attempt at dieting. Some of the patients may have been obese, but many have only fears or fantasies of becoming fat.

4. The patient often has a hostile-dependent relationship with her mother, and there may be an overtly seductive quality in the father-daughter relationship.

5. During preadolescence the patients are often overconscientious, energetic and high achievers.

6. There are usually conflicts around emancipation from the parents which reflect the underlying difficulties in separation-individuation.

7. There may be significant difficulties in heterosexual relationships with many activities and athletic preoccupations being substituted for dates or social interaction.

8. The onset may be related to menarche or to a traumatic conflict in the psychosexual area.

HISTORY FROM THE PARENTS:

1. The initial examination should usually be done with both parents being seen together, but separately from the patient.

2. The relationship between the patient and the parents, especially the mother, should be evaluated. There is often a strong, overcontrolling attitude on the part of the mother toward the patient.

3. Parents may overvalue slimness and physical attractiveness.

4. Parents may be highly invested in issues concerning food, for example, calorie content, preparation, "eating everything on your plate, " etc. Some parents may even be engaged in occupations related to food preparation.

HISTORY FROM THE CHILD:

1. Initially, the child should be examined without the parents present. Subsequent evaluation may include the parents if this can be tolerated by the child.

2. Patients often appear preoccupied or irritable and have difficulty talking about their feelings.

3. Highly symbolic meanings are often attached to body weight and contours. Pregnancy fantasies may occur.

4. Self-destruction or unconscious suicidal implications of the failure to eat may be involved in the refusal to eat.

5. Patients may have a distorted self-concept, with failure to be in touch with body sensations or functions.

6. Some patients may have a normal appetite but refuse to eat from a fear of digestive or swallowing discomfort.

7. Semistarvation may serve as a form of self-punishment and purification related to underlying guilt feelings.

PSYCHOLOGICAL SIGNS AND SYMPTOMS:

1. Loss of psychological appetite

2. Denial of physical hunger

3. Aversion to food or peculiar food preferences

4. Activity is most often strikingly maintained in the presence of severe weight loss.

5. Food binges followed by self-induced vomiting

6. Mixed hysterical and phobic states in which eating may have strong sexual implications

7. Obsessive-compulsive states in which eating may raise fears of dirt in the food or contamination

8. Schizophrenic or borderline psychotic states in which eating may lead to fears of poisoning

PHYSICAL SIGNS AND SYMPTOMS:

1. Severe weight loss

2. Hypoproteinemia, with edema at times

3. Emaciation and pallor

4. Amenorrhea. About 50% of the patients develop amenorrhea before losing weight and the other 50% develop amenorrhea as the malnutrition progresses.

5. Lowered body temperature, pulse rate and blood pressure

6. Dryness of the skin and brittleness of the nails

7. Flat or occasionally diabetic blood sugar curves

8. Hypercholesterolemia

9. Hypokalemia secondary to self-induced vomiting

10. Constipation

DIFFERENTIAL DIAGNOSIS:

1. Chronic diseases, especially granulomatous disease of the small bowel or inflammation of the small or large bowel

2. Neoplasms

3. Occult infections

4. Pathological lesions of the esophagus, stomach or duodenum

5. Depression associated with organic illness, such as pancre-

atic disorders or liver disease

6. Primary depressive illness

7. Anterior pituitary insufficiency, Simmonds' disease

IMMEDIATE TREATMENT:

1. A complete medical evaluation is indicated to rule out organic causes for weight loss.

2. If body weight falls below 50% of ideal weight, a combined medical and psychological approach is mandatory. Tube feeding or a hyperalimentation line may be necessary to provide calories if the patient refuses to eat. This treatment can often be carried out on a general pediatric inpatient setting.

3. Seriously disturbed patients with schizophrenic or borderline psychotic states should have their initial treatment in a psychiatric, inpatient setting (Galdston, 1974).

4. Less disturbed patients can often be treated as outpatients, either individually or in family sessions, using appropriate psychotherapeutic modalities (Bruch, 1970).

5. Underlying conflicts between family members involving eating, sexuality and control should be explored (Liebman, et al., 1974).

6. Psychoactive medication may be indicated in the more seriously disturbed patients.

7. Behavior modification approaches, with careful attention to rewarding weight gain, are nearly always indicated (Blinder, et al., 1970).

FOLLOW-UP TREATMENT:

1. With patients who require hospitalization in a pediatric or psychiatric unit, the discharge plans should include consideration of the following:

   a) Placement of the patient out of the home

   b) Careful follow-up by the involved pediatrician and psychiatrist or psychologist concerning post-hospitalization treatment plans for (1) the patient if she is to be living away from home or (2) for the patient and her family if the patient is to return home

c) Public health nurse support to help the patient and the family continue the treatment plans

d) Ongoing communication among all parties involved in the patient's treatment

e) Rehospitalization if progressive weight loss recurs

2. For patients not requiring hospitalization, close communication must be maintained between the patient, her family and the professional staff involved in her treatment.

: :

CHILD ABUSE

GENERAL COMMENTS:

The term "battered child syndrome" was coined in 1962 by Kempe (Kempe, et al. , 1962). It encompasses any condition injurious to the child's physical or emotional health that has been inflicted by parents, guardians or other caretakers, or has resulted from their lack of reasonable care and protection. The categories of child abuse include physical abuse, sexual abuse, emotional abuse and neglect of medical care and safety. Approximately 10% of injuries seen in a hospital emergency room, in children under 5 years of age, have been inflicted by a caretaker (Holter and Friedman, 1968). Physical abuse is the second most frequent cause of death in the age group one month to six months of age.

HISTORY:

History obtained from parents frequently includes the following points:

1. Repeated beatings or severe deprivation of either parent as a child

2. Past record of serious mental illness or repeated difficulties of either parent with the law

3. Severe prenatal or postpartum depression in the mother

4. Violent temper outbursts in either parent against the child or others

5. Serious marital discord or generally chaotic life-style

6. Family crisis (job loss, change in residence, acute illness in the child, intractable crying, death in the family, birth of a sibling or discovery of an unwanted pregnancy)

7. Social isolation (lack of lifelines, close friends or social life)

8. Inappropriate, rigid standards of child behavior (expectations of performance beyond the capacity for obedience or intolerance of normal annoying behavior)

9. Unwanted or unrewarding child (premature, illegitimate, adopted, neonatal complications causing prolonged separation or defiant misbehavior)

10. Delay in seeking medical care, failure to get routine care, or seeking care from several facilities

11. Repeated suspicious injuries or accidents

12. Role reversal (parents expecting their children to meet their needs and make them feel better)

13. Poor match in temperament between child and caretaker (Thomas, et al. , 1968; Thomas and Chess, 1977)

EXAMINATION OF THE PARENTS OR CARETAKERS:

Parents should be evaluated together and separately, and examination should include the following items:

1. Parents' capacity to see likeable attributes in the child and to see the child as a separate individual

2. Parents' capacity to relieve each other or call for help in a crisis

3. Stability of marital, occupational, and living conditions

4. Father's support of mother and involvement in the child's care

5. Parents' ability to have fun together and share personal interests and hobbies

6. Parents' role models when growing up

7. Parents' coping abilities (capacity to plan and understand the need for adjustment as a result of the new baby)

8. Child's health and development

9. Complete history of present injury

10. Previous history of unexplained injuries or inability to explain present injury

11. Different description of injury from each parent

12. Contradictions between the history offered and the physical findings (the history of a minor accident and the findings of a major injury)

13. Alleged self-injury in an infant

14. Blaming a third party for an injury or accident

15. Parents' psychiatric history and present mental status (evaluate for psychosis, drug or alcohol abuse, severe depression or sociopathy) (Steele and Pollock, 1974; Coppolillo, 1975)

EXAMINATION OF THE CHILD:

1. Examine infants and children under age 3 with the parents, in order to note the parent-child interaction

2. Interview the child over age 3 with the parents and then individually, in a diagnostic play interview

3. Do a complete physical, neurological and developmental examination

4. X-ray the skull and long bones, photograph the injuries, and screen for bleeding disorders

5. Assess for speech delays (Blager and Martin 1976)

6. Evaluate for unusual compliance and efforts to please adults

7. Assess for inhibition of affect

SIGNS AND SYMPTOMS
(Schmitt and Kempe, 1975):

1. Bruises, welts, and scars: These are usually located on the buttocks and lower back. Finger and thumb prints, hand-prints, and bruising of the upper lip and frenulum may be seen. Human bite marks, loop marks from a doubled-over cord or rope, lash marks from a belt, tree branch or hard-edged ruler, and choke and gag marks also may be seen. Most accidents cause bruises on only one body surface. Bruises on multiple body planes usually have been inflicted, unless there is a history of tumbling accidents plus associated abrasions or contusions on the elbows, knees and shoulders.

2. Burns: The most commonly inflicted burn is caused by a cigarette. This causes circular, punched-out areas of similar size which are found most often on the palms, soles or abdomen. Dry contact burns result from a child being held against a radiator, heating grate, hot iron or other hot dry surface. Hot water burns or dunking burns occur when the parent holds the child's thighs against the abdomen and dunks the buttocks and perineum into a bucket of scalding water. The hands and feet are spared.

3. Eye injuries: These include acute hyphema (blood in the anterior chamber), dislocated lenses and detached retinas.

4. Central nervous system injuries: The child may present with skull fracture, coma, convulsions, increased intra-cranial pressure and retinal hemorrhages. Subdural hema-toma may be caused by a blow to the head or from violent whiplash-type shaking injuries. Subgaleal hematoma may result from vigorous hair pulling, especially at the site of a tight braid. Cephalohematoma, epidural hematoma, and spinal cord injuries may also result from trauma to these areas.

5. Abdominal visceral injuries: These may be caused by the force of a punch or blow to the child's abdomen. The child presents with recurrent vomiting, abdominal distention, absent bowel sound or localized tenderness.

6. Bone injuries: Fractures of long bones, fingers and toes, skull, ribs, and pelvis may be seen on X-ray.

DIFFERENTIAL DIAGNOSIS:

1. Bleeding disorders

2. Hyperactivity combined with accident proneness

3. Neurological disorders that mimic trauma

4. Developmental delays or deviations

5. Rare bone disorder (osteogenesis imperfecta, infantile cortical hyperostosis, scurvy, syphilis, and neoplasms)

IMMEDIATE TREATMENT:

1. Hospitalize suspected cases (Helfer, 1974)

2. Treat the child's injuries or malnutrition

3. Obtain all necessary laboratory tests and X-rays

4. Maintain a helping, supportive approach to parents

5. Tell parents the diagnosis and the legal obligation to report it

6. Examine all siblings within 12 hours

7. Involve the parents in the child's hospital care and observe parent-child interactions

8. Report the suspected abuse to the appropriate child protective agency within 24 hours

9. Submit an official written report within 48 hours

10. Obtain hospital social service consultation within 48 hours

11. Provide crisis intervention, psychiatric consultation if necessary

12. Appoint an attorney to represent the abused child as his counsel and guardian ad litem.

FOLLOW-UP TREATMENT:

1. Make weekly visits for medical follow-up until a stable set-

ting is achieved

2. Assess the safety of the child's home

3. Provide a multidisciplinary team to consider legal decisions regarding the return of the child to the natural parents, temporary foster home placement or termination of parental rights and to make a recommendation to the appropriate court

4. Arrange psychiatric follow-up for the parent or parents

5. Provide psychiatric follow-up for the child

6. Make available to every family suspected of child abuse lay therapists, mothering aides, homemakers, parents anonymous groups, telephone hotlines, day care centers, crisis nurseries, child-rearing group sessions, and vocational rehabilitation services

7. Arrange for a court review to be conducted in 6-12 months

: :

CHILDHOOD PSYCHOSES

GENERAL COMMENTS:

There is much confusion and disagreement regarding the diagnosis of childhood psychoses. Some attempts have been made to classify childhood psychoses on the basis of etiological considerations, and thus, there are classifications such as early infantile autism and symbiotic psychosis. Other attempts have been made to classify these psychoses on the basis of ego functions or ego deficits (Beres, 1956), and from these attempts come terms such as the child with atypical ego development (Rank, 1955). Finally, attempts to classify these disorders on the basis of phenomenological or descriptive considerations have resulted in terms such as schizophreniform psychosis, hysterical psychosis, folie a deux, manic depressive psychosis and Heller's disease.

There is much discussion as to whether certain types of childhood psychosis are indeed similar in any important way to other types. For example, many feel (Rutter, 1968; Miller, 1973) that so-called early infantile autism is an entirely separate entity from the other childhood psychoses. Another im-

portant question is whether childhood psychosis is any more
than superficially similar to adult psychosis. It is known that
the continuities between childhood psychoses and adult psychoses are few, and that children with childhood psychoses are
very different when grown up from other adults with the adult-
type schizophrenias.

Although a relatively rare illness in children (probably less
than 1 in 1000) as compared to adults (1 in 50 to 1 in 100), childhood psychosis presents as a child psychiatric emergency much
more frequently than usually expected from its incidence.

In general, psychotic states in children are characterized by
marked deviations or delays in many areas of development.
Delays or deviations in these areas are: (1) unrelatedness to
people; (2) peculiar relatedness to the nonhuman environment;
(3) unevenness of the level of emotional maturation; (4) unevenness in the development of various so-called ego functions, including perception, sensory-motor functions and intelligence;
and (5) deficits in the development of a sense of self and a sense
of self as separate and individual.

Although differential diagnosis is difficult, several somewhat
distinct subgroups have emerged over recent years and will be
briefly discussed in turn. These subgroups are:

A. Childhood Schizophrenia
B. Early Infantile Autism
C. Symbiotic Psychosis or Interactional Psychosis
D. Schizophreniform Psychosis
E. Manic-Depressive Illness
F. Hysterical Psychosis
G. Folie a Deux

Whenever a diagnosis of childhood psychosis is considered, a
number of psychotic and nonpsychotic organic conditions must
be ruled out. These include deafness, aphasia, mental retardation, and acute and chronic brain syndromes.

CHILDHOOD SCHIZOPHRENIA

At one time, nearly all childhood psychoses were lumped together under this single classification. Gradually, various distinct entities have been removed from this general category.
The most difficult remaining differentiation is between childhood schizophrenia and early infantile autism. After the enti-

ties of early infantile autism and symbiotic psychosis have been removed, the remaining somewhat heterogeneous group can be called childhood schizophrenia. The exact diagnosis of childhood schizophrenia may be difficult to establish. The following 15 points are Hingtgen and Bryson's (1972) expansion of the 9 points outlined by the British Working Party (Creak, 1964), and are considered to be among the most important characteristics of children with childhood schizophrenia:

1. Extreme self-isolation, aloofness or withdrawal noticeable in infancy, including unresponsiveness to the mother and unresponsiveness to gestures or expression of affection

2. Lack or avoidance of eye contact: looking through or past people

3. Repetitive and peculiar use of toys and objects in an inappropriate manner and/or similar repetitive and peculiar body motions, such as incessant rocking, dependence on seemingly self-imposed rituals

4. Abnormal speech development:

   a) Failure to develop speech
   b) Speech disappears at an early age
   c) Limited speech or echolalia without communication
   d) Pronominal reversal
   e) Abnormal use and comprehension of language
   f) Compulsive, excessive, meaningless and bizarre speech

5. Insistence on sameness (in objects and their placement, as well as in routines)

6. More attention paid to objects than to people

7. Use of people as objects or tools

8. Seeming insensitivity to pain

9. Self-mutilation, head banging

10. Laughing or smiling, crying or tantrums for no apparent reason

11. Preoccupation with bizarre and elaborate systems or fantasies, carrying strong positive or negative affect

12. Retardation with islets of normal functioning: unusual abilities, for example, rote memory, music, geography, numbers

13. Abnormal responses to stimuli; hypo- or hyper-sensitivity, especially to sound

14. Abnormal fears or lack of appropriate sense of fear

15. Extreme negativism; no imitation of others, except in speech

DIFFERENTIAL DIAGNOSIS:

These 15 points include many items that would lead to a diagnosis of early infantile autism; however, many workers believe that early infantile autism is a separate entity (Rutter, 1972).

Childhood schizophrenia, of an early onset type, can be differentiated from early infantile autism by the following characteristics (De Myer, et al. , 1971):

1. In childhood schizophrenia, islands of normal relatedness and even excessive dependency are seen against a background of emotional withdrawal; whereas in early infantile autism, extreme emotional withdrawal and aloofness are observed.

2. In childhood schizophrenia, some speech with speech abnormalities for communication is seen; whereas in early infantile autism, a lack of communicative speech is observed.

Later onset (age 7 and older) childhood schizophrenia can be distinguished from early infantile autism by the following characteristics:

1. Relapses and remissions characterize later onset childhood schizophrenia, while the course of early infantile autism is more nearly continuous.

2. Later onset childhood schizophrenia more closely resembles adult schizophrenia with a greater incidence of blocking, loose associations, hallucinations, delusions, blunting of affect and disturbance of mood (Kolvin, et al. , 1971).

3. Schizophrenia is relatively frequent (10%) in the parents and

siblings of children with late onset childhood schziophrenia but is no more common than in the general population among the parents and siblings of children with early infantile autism.

TREATMENT:

Treatment and treatment considerations regarding childhood schizophrenia are similar to those of early infantile autism. Treatment for the two similar, but probably distinct entities, is discussed in the following section (see p. 46).

EARLY INFANTILE AUTISM

GENERAL COMMENTS AND DEFINITION:

In 1943, Kanner described a group of children with the following characteristics:

1. Extreme self-isolation including:

   a) A preference for objects over people
   b) Avoidance of eye contact
   c) Failure to cuddle or mold to the mother's body
   d) At times, a trance-like expression
   e) No anticipatory behavior on the approach of the mother
   f) A bright, alert-appearing expression
   g) Early feeding and sleeping difficulties
   h) Poor language development including:
      (1) Pronominal reversal (me exchanged for you)
      (2) Echolalia (repeating the last few words heard)

2. An anxiously obsessive desire for the preservation of sameness including:

   a) A concern for incomplete or damaged objects or surfaces such as broken toys, cracks in the floor or walls, burnt out lightbulbs, etc.
   b) Obsessive bedtime and feeding rituals

3. Motor behaviors and rituals including:

   a) Unusually skillful manipulation of objects
   b) Rocking in a rhythmic way
   c) Twirling

4. Special isolated skills or abilities such as:

   a) Unusual musical abilities
   b) Ability to calculate quickly
   c) Unusual feats of memory

5. The use of proximal (smelling, tasting, feeling) receptors, rather than distal (hearing, seeing) receptors in exploring their world

FAMILY HISTORY AND EXAMINATION OF THE
CHILD AND FAMILY:

1. Parents of autistic children were originally described as "refrigerator parents" who had difficulty in relating warmly to their children and were more interested in things than in people (Kanner, 1943). This description has not been verified as being specific or causitive in early infantile autism (Rutter, et al. , 1967).

2. Other family characteristics that have been noted, but may be considered as incompletely verified are:

   a) The child's withdrawal in response to negative emotions on the part of the mother, and a subsequent sense of helplessness on the part of the child (Bettelheim, 1967)

   b) An impairment of the integrating, synthesizing and organizing functions of the ego, as a result of the infant's inability "to utilize the mother as a complement to and organizer of its maturation" during its early phases of life (Mahler and Furer, 1972)

   c) Overt maternal depression (Reiser, 1963; O'Gorman, 1970; Szurek and Berlin, 1973; Tustin, 1972)

3. A number of studies supports the idea of a disorder in central nervous system maturation or development as being at least highly contributory to infantile autism:

   a) Fish and her co-workers felt that "uneven neurological development, characterized by unusual combinations of retardation and precocity "could lead an infant to be vulnerable to early childhood schizophrenia or early infantile autism (Fish, et al. , 1966).

   b) Others have proposed a variety of sensory and sensory-motor integration disorders (Reichler and Schopler, 1971; Ornitz and Ritvo, 1968; Birch and Hertzig, 1967).

c) Genetic influences have been implicated, and it has been noted that 11 of 14 monozygotic pairs of twins have been concordant for infantile autism (Rimland, 1964).

d) Numerous associated anomalies have been noted to exist with unusual frequency in infantile autism. Among these are the following:

    (1) Perinatal difficulties
    (2) Neurological "soft signs"
    (3) Abnormal EEGs
    (4) Below average IQ
    (5) Perceptual disorders
    (6) Language disorders
    (7) Abnormal neurochemical status
    (8) Unusual sensitivities

TREATMENT AND LONG-TERM PROGNOSIS:

1. Numerous modalities of treatment are currently being used with autistic children and children with childhood schizophrenia, and no methods of treatment have met with complete success. However, the prognosis is thought to be more favorable now than in previous follow-up studies (Eisenberg, 1956/ Eisenberg, 1957).

2. Residential or day psychiatric treatment should always be considered. The emphasis in the treatment should include extensive language and cognitive stimulation in an intensive therapeutic milieu. An aggressive effort to "break through the autistic shell" by an individual child psychotherapist and staff members within the milieu is an important element in treatment.

3. Psychopharmacological treatment may be a useful adjunct in controlling destructive or self-mutilating behavior but is unlikely to be effective in altering the core symptomatology.

4. Electroconvulsive therapy has not been shown as beneficial to autistic or schizophrenic children and should never be used.

5. The best predictors of a successful outcome of treatment are:

a) Level of language development (Eisenberg, 1956)
b) Intelligence (DeMyer, et al., 1973; Rutter, et al., 1967)
c) Severity of symptomatology
d) Attendance at school for at least two years (Rutter, et al., 1967)

6. Counselling with parents and the use of parents as "auxillary therapists" have been found especially useful by Schopler and Reichler (1971). In their treatment program, they view the autistic or schizophrenic child as a child who has constitutional deficits, and treatment is geared toward improving specific language, cognitive and perceptual skills. They utilize operant conditioning, special educational methods and at times, psychoactive medications.

SYMBIOTIC PSYCHOSIS OR INTERACTIONAL PSYCHOSIS

1. This type of childhood psychosis was first described by Margaret Mahler (1952) and has subsequently been described by others (Furer, 1964; Bergman, 1971) It is characterized by the following description:

   a) An extremely close attachment to the mother often involving clinging and close physical contact

   b) Poor language development and possibly immature language that is understood only by the mother

   c) Extreme anxiety with a primitive, panic-stricken quality on the part of the child when separation of mother and child is attempted

   d) Anxiety on the part of the mother and prominent fantasies of harm coming to the child when separation is attempted

   e) General immaturity in all phases of development

   f) A failure of the child to appreciate himself/herself as separate and individual from the mother

   g) At times, special intense attachments to personal objects belonging to the mother (hairbrush, handkerchief)

2. The cause of this type of childhood psychosis is presumed to be a failure of negotiation of the separation-individuation phase of child development (Mahler, et al., 1975; Mahler and Furer,

1960) during approximately the period from 6 months to 3 years of age.

3. The first year of life is usually normal by history, with the exception of an unusually close mother-child relationship.

4. Treatment usually involves long-term psychotherapy with both the mother and the child. Attention is focused on the nature of the relationship, the fears of each around separation, the hostile and aggressive fantasies of each toward the other, and the hopeful accomplishment of separation and individuation on the part of the child. Usually during the beginning phases of psychotherapy, the mother and child must be seen together because separation is impossible to accomplish.

5. Prognosis is usually favorable, given good cooperation by both parents. Attention to the father's role in the illness is important. In particular, the mother's appropriate turning to the father for gratification and support instead of depending on the child should be facilitated by the therapist.

6. A failure of outpatient psychotherapy may necessitate residential or day psychiatric hospitalization.

7. Medication is only indicated for the control of target symptoms such as self-destructive behavior or insomnia.

SCHIZOPHRENIFORM PSYCHOSIS

This diagnostic entity has been described by Jordan and Prugh (1971) and is defined by the following characteristics, as noted in the 1966 report on Psychopathological Disorders in Childhood (Group for the Advancement of Psychiatry, 1966):

1. The onset is usually between the ages of six and twelve with no evidence of an earlier psychosis.

2. There is a gradual appearance of neurotic symptoms first, followed by marked and primitive denial and projection, looseness of associations, low frustration tolerance, hypochondriacal tendencies, and intense temper outbursts.

3. In some cases, marked withdrawal, autistic behaviors, emotional aloofness, intense involvement in fantasy, extreme anxiety, marked phobias and distorted reality testing may

be seen.

4. Bizarre behavior, including stereotyped motor patterns such as whirling and rocking, wild aggressive or self-mutilating outbursts, suicidal threats, somatic delusions, ideas of reference, and paranoid thinking are frequently present.

5. Regression is not usually as pronounced as in the adult psychoses, and true hallucinations are not usually seen.

6. The prognosis for a complete recovery from the first episode is good, which helps to differentiate this type from other forms of childhood psychoses. Crystallization into the adult subtypes of schizophrenia seldom occurs.

7. Treatment which included a brief hospitalization followed by one to two years of weekly outpatient treatment was shown to be effective (Jordan and Prugh, 1971).

MANIC-DEPRESSIVE ILLNESS

DEFINITION:

Mania is a phase of what is now called bipolar illness. In unipolar illness patients show only depression. In bipolar illness patients have a family history of mania, episodes of both mania and depression, an augmenting pattern in their cortical-evoked potentials, and an earlier onset than unipolar patients. When bipolars are depressed, they tend to have what is known as a retarded type of depression, in that they show less pacing, less overt expressions of anger, and fewer somatic complaints than unipolars (Kessler, 1975).

GENERAL COMMENTS:

1. Manic-depressive illness is relatively uncommon, affecting about 1.5% of the population.

2. Two women are affected for every man, so the incidence in women is 2% and in men, 1%.

3. If a patient has one manic episode, he/she has a 75% chance for recurrence of mania and a 95% chance for the occurrence of depression. Thus, only 5% of manic-depressive patients show recurrent mania alone.

4. Gilbert pointed out that a person in a fully developed manic state is "as easy to identify as a hurricane or a tidal wave. He comes on like . . . a banjo-strumming, derby hat-wearing, tap-dancing gorilla with a light-up bow tie, arising from a trap door in the floor" (Gilbert, 1969). Despite this whimsical description, and despite the fact that Kraeplin (1921) noted that the greatest frequency of first attacks was between the fifteenth and the twentieth year, mania has been seen largely as a disease of adulthood and one causing some difficulty in diagnosis (Horowitz, 1977). Manic-depressive illness is seen infrequently in children and for a period of time was thought to be nonexistent. Anthony and Scott (1960) could not find anyone under age eleven who met their ten criteria for an actual episode of mania.

5. More recently, Feinstein and Wolpert (1973), and then McKnew and co-workers (1974), reported on cases of juvenile manic-depressive illness or hypomania in children. Winokur and his co-workers (1971) noted that one-third of their sample of bipolar patients became ill before the age of 20.

6. While it has been argued that childhood and adolescent onset manic-depressive illness might be a different disorder than the adult onset type, Carlson and co-workers (1977) found that early age of onset was not a factor in the course and prognosis of manic-depressive illness. Their study compared patients with onset of illness before age twenty to those with onset after age forty-five.

HISTORY AND FAMILY BACKGROUND:

1. Some authors (Cohen, et al. , 1954; Cohen, 1975) have felt that the infancy of the manic-depressive patient is normal, that the childhood is conforming and repressed, and that the manic episode occurs later in life.

2. Arieti (1974) feels that the manic patient is born in a home which is accepting and caring for the first year. Then in the second year, the mother makes many demands on the child. He receives care and affection only when he accepts the high expectations placed on him. This sharp transition may be brought on by the parents' own dissatisfactions and resentments, by displacement through the birth of a younger sibling, or by a sharp transition from breast-feeding to feeding from a cup. In some patients, the abrupt change may take place somewhat later, but it usually occurs in the preschool years. Some support for this hypothesis is found in

the fact that the manic-depressive tends to be firstborn and therefore, more likely to be displaced.

3. Arieti (1974) also notes that the family is often a member of a "marginal" group because of religious or ethnic status. The child learns to have high expectations in order to "rescue" the family from its lowered status. Some support for this concept is seen in the fact that people of Jewish and Irish ethnic groups are said to have a higher than average incidence of manic-depressive illness.

4. Later, the child senses that being like his parents is too difficult because of their high expectations, and to compensate he turns to other adults with whom he identifies to an exaggerated degree. Therefore, there is no single significant adult to whom the child can relate in a meaningful way. This identification with many adults can lead to a personality organization which is active and friendly, but which on closer examination, is seen to be superficial. Sometimes these traits are so exaggerated that the patient can be considered hypomanic or sociopathic.

5. There is strong evidence for a genetic contribution to manic-depressive illness. The average concordance for monozygotic twins is 68% and for same-sexed dizygotic twins, 23%. Parents, children and siblings of manic-depressive patients have about a 15% chance of developing an affective disorder. Some findings are suggestive of an X-linked dominant mode of inheritance, but more recent studies would suggest a polygenic mode of inheritance (Kessler, 1975).

SIGNS AND SYMPTOMS:

1. Characteristically, the manic patient presents with elation accompanied by an increase in psychomotor behavior:

   a) The patient's affect may be either elation or irritability. Carlson (1978) has noted that irritability seems more common in adolescent mania.

   b) The increase in motor behavior may be manifested by a need to do things quickly, to make increasing numbers of long-distance calls, to pace, to travel great distances to visit relatives, or to run away. The patient commonly reports a decreased need for sleep and food (eating on the run).

c) Cognitively, the patient has a flight of ideas (racing thoughts) resulting in pressured speech and distractibility. These are commonly associated with a grandiosity in which the patient feels he/she can accomplish, or is about to accomplish great things, yet does not finish what he/she starts. This state may progress to the point of frank delusions. Less commonly, the patient may be paranoid. Usually, this manifests itself in the patient's delusional belief that persons are attempting to block some grandiose scheme he/she may have; or he/she may hear voices calling to him/her to accomplish his/her scheme.

2. Relationships are characterized by a superficial warmth and gaiety and have been well described by Cohen (1975).

a) In hypomania, the patient is friendly and overly warm, then uninvitedly intimate and overly personal. Just under the surface are impatience and intolerance when wishes are not immediately gratified. The patient is impulsive and uses poor judgment but dismisses errors as trivial.

b) In acute mania, all of the previously mentioned motor, affective, cognitive and relationship qualities are intensified so that propriety and convention are lost. The patient teases and jokes. Puns give way to clang associations. Good humor quickly becomes vicious anger, and strong verbal attacks occur when the patient is confronted. Unless verbal and/or physical restraints are applied, every thought is followed by action. The patient is now clearly psychotic in the sense that he/she has lost control over his/her behavior.

c) Delirious mania is the most severe form of mania and is quite rare. Motor activity is constant and without purpose. Affect rapidly fluctuates between anger and sorrow. Cognitively, the patient is delirious with disorientation and confusion. Hallucinations and delusions are common. Relationships are impossible. Incontinence of urine and feces may also occur. In earlier years, before adequate treatment was available, death sometimes occurred.

DIAGNOSIS AND DIFFERENTIAL DIAGNOSIS:

1. Since an effective treatment now exists for manic episodes, this diagnosis must be considered in the evaluation of any disturbed adolescent.

2. One set of diagnostic criteria in common use is that of
Feighner and his co-workers (1972). All of the following,
are required for a diagnosis of mania:

a) Euphoria or irritability

b) At least three of the following:

    (1) Hyperactivity, including motor activity, social ac-
tivity and sexual activity
    (2) Push of speech: the pressure to keep talking
    (3) Flight of ideas: racing thoughts
    (4) Grandiosity: sometimes of delusional proportions
    (5) Decreased sleep
    (6) Distractibility

c) A psychiatric illness lasting at least two weeks without any of
the following preexisting psychiatric conditions, such as:

    (1) Schizophrenia
    (2) Anxiety, phobic, obsessive-compulsive and hysteri-
cal neuroses
    (3) Drug dependence, including alcoholism
    (4) Antisocial personality
    (5) Sexual deviation including sexual orientation distur-
bance
    (6) Mental retardation
    (7) Organic brain syndrome

3. In adolescents and children, it is important to exclude the hyperkinetic reaction. The manic patient and the hyperkinetic child
have, in common, hyperactivity, a decreased need for
sleep and distractibility. However, the hyperkinetic child
will have a long history of these symptoms, while the manic
patient's symptoms will usually be of recent onset. The hyperkinetic child is also likely to have associated learning
disabilities which are rarely present in the manic patient.
The hyperkinetic child or adolescent will almost always lack
the grandiosity and flight of ideas of the manic patient.
Overall, the comparison suggests two automobiles, both
with their engines racing. The hyperkinetic child seems to
have some teeth missing in his gears so that everything is
done with a jerking unevenness. The manic patient is smooth

but just too fast for the road conditions.

4. Previously, it was felt that patients with schizophrenia could be distinguished from those suffering manic-depressive illness by the presence of delusions, and especially hallucinations. Now, it has been pointed out that 20-25% of manic-depressive patients will have delusions, hallucinations, or even first-rank Schneiderian symptoms of schizophrenia, such as thought intrusion or broadcasting. This complicates the diagnostic picture considerably. Since manic-depressive patients, in contrast to patients with schizophrenia do not have a downhill course, even more caution should be used in making a diagnosis of schizophrenia in patients with delusions or hallucinations. When present, the manic patient's delusions and hallucinations will center around his/her grandiose schemes.

5. As noted earlier, 95% of all manic patients will have an episode of depression, and these are commonly of the retarded type with early morning awakening, weight loss, gradual onset and painfully depressed affect. Since this type of depression is relatively uncommon in adolescence, its presentation should raise the index of suspicion for manic-depressive illness.

6. This author has evaluated manic adolescents who initially presented as a toxic response to marijuana (Hebert, 1978). Horowitz (1977) described marijuana as a preceding factor in mania in two of four cases he presented but did not offer comment. It is difficult to ascertain whether this correlation represents simply the nearly universal frequency of marijuana use among adolescents or an abnormal response to a mild euphoriant. The precipitation of mania in adults by tricyclic antidepressants is well known and can be hypothesized for cocaine and amphetamines as well.

EXAMINATION OF THE CHILD:

1. It is important to examine the child in an area free of distraction because of the distractibility inherent in the manic phase.

2. If impulsiveness and psychomotor agitation are pronounced, a secure room may be necessary to prevent runaway.

3. Structure, and calm, firmly made requests for cooperation can help facilitate the interview.

IMMEDIATE TREATMENT:

1. The adolescent's propensity for action, coupled with an illness that increases motor activity and impairs judgment,
   make hospitalization necessary in the initial stage of treatment for acute mania:

   a) The patient needs to be told quietly and firmly what is
      about to happen and what he/she needs to do to partici-
      pate in the treatment.

   b) In contrast to the families of disoriented, organically,
      psychotic patients, the family of the manic patient is less
      often helpful. Family members frequently have indulged
      the patient and, though only minutes before they have
      brought the patient in to enter the hospital, they may have
      a change of heart or back down and acquiesce to yet an-
      other last demand of the patient.

   c) A secure room may be necessary to control agitation and
      a tendency to run.

   d) Major tranquilizers may be necessary to control behav-
      ior during the first days on the ward while lithium reach-
      es therapeutic levels (see Chapter V, p. 153).

2. Bipolar patients who present in the depressed state also
   represent a crisis and often need hospitalization:

   a) The presence of a severe depressed mood, worse in the
      morning, with psychomotor retardation, serious weight
      loss and early morning or middle of the night awakening
      is unusual enough to warrant suspicion of a biological
      depressive process even though a family history of manic-
      depressive illness is not obtained.

   b) Even those adolescents who later prove to have bipolar
      illness will usually present with a mood that is a mixture
      of depression, anxiety and the feeling that things are not
      right. In addition to malaise, they will have numerous
      physical complaints, mostly referable to the gastroin-
      testinal tract: nausea, a feeling of being choked up, vague
      abdominal discomfort, constipation and fatigue. Motor
      activity is characterized by restlessness.

   c) Every patient should be questioned for suicidal ideation.
      Thoughts of a dramatic death are common in adolescents,

but any suicidal plans are an indication for hospitalization. High speed driving in male adolescents and promiscuity with multiple partners in female adolescents often contain hidden suicidal ideation.

d) Treatment can be initiated cautiously on an outpatient basis if the physician feels he/she has an alliance with the patient, <u>except</u> when there are suicidal plans, lack of supportive environment or the history of a previous manic attack. In the latter case, the danger of suicide is so high that hospitalization is needed.

FOLLOW-UP TREATMENT:

1. The manic patient will need the following:

   a) A physical exam, thyroid (T_3 T_4) and kidney function studies (BUN, creatinine) must be performed to ensure that there are no contra-indications to the use of lithium.

   b) Lithium carbonate is begun in divided doses with the therapeutic dose determined by the patient's response, side-effects and laboratory indications of blood level (see Chapter V, p. 154).

   c) Initial psychotherapy includes support, clear limit setting and active participation in the treatment plan.

2. The depressed bipolar patient will need the following:

   a) A physical exam must be performed to be certain that the patient does not suffer from narrow angle glaucoma or heart disease which would predispose to arrhythmias from tricyclic antidepressants.

   b) Initially, hospitalization for a one- to two-week period without medication is indicated. Most adolescents with vegetative signs of depression will lose these, as well as some of their depressed affect, during this time period. If, at the end of this time, there is still a middle of the night or early morning sleep disturbance and if the patient has not regained some appetite, tricyclic medications can be given (see Chapter V, p. 152).

   c) Psychotherapy is begun on admission. Since the depressed patient has difficulty relating, sessions are kept short and frequent, with the therapist being an active participant.

3. In long-term, follow-up therapy, as he/she returns to the baseline state, the bipolar patient comes to see the therapist as a powerful, but friendly, supportive figure. The patient has an opportunity to build an identification with a single significant adult. Transference reactions are used to point out to the patient how his/her self-esteem is built on the approval of others, rather than being internally based (Cohen, 1975).

HYSTERICAL PSYCHOSIS

Hysterical psychosis is differentiated from the other psychoses of childhood by the following characteristics:

1. The symptoms, usually consisting of delusions, hallucinations, feelings of depersonalization and disturbed behavior, are of a particularly bizarre and florid nature.

2. The onset is usually rapid, and a clear precipitant can be identified.

3. The incidence is greatest in adolescent girls with a preexisting hysterical personality type.

4. The delusions often do not meet the criteria of incorrigibility (Siomopoulis, 1971) in that they are more amenable to correction through reality confrontation by the examiner.

5. Clearing of the psychotic episode is often rapid following resolution of the precipitating situation (Hollender and Hirsch, 1964).

6. Recurrence and/or residual deficit is unusual.

7. Areas of ego functioning not involved in the specific delusions and/or hallucinations are relatively unimpaired.

8. Brief separation from, resolution of, or relief from the precipitating environmental stress is usually indicated as a part of treatment. A brief hospitalization of one week to ten days is usually sufficient.

FOLIE A DEUX

GENERAL COMMENTS AND DEFINITION:

1. This term was coined by Lasegue and Falret (1877) and applies to a psychosis shared by two persons, one of whom is regarded as the dominant or inducing partner and the other as the submissive partner who colludes. This condition is seen infrequently in adults and even less frequently in children, which is surprising considering that normal children are suggestible, easily influenced and dependent on their parents.

2. Coleman outlined the following necessary conditions for folie a deux to occur (Coleman and Last, 1939):

   a) The inductor must have a strong motivation to have his/her delusional ideas accepted by the passive member and must even be willing to modify them to achieve this.

   b) The delusions must not be so idiosyncratic as to prohibit personal involvement by the other person.

   c) The passive partner must be a suggestible, possible hysterical person whose wishes would in some way be fulfilled by the delusional system.

   d) The dominant and passive members must have lived together in close association for some time.

3. The actual psychosis usually takes the form of a fixed delusion, usually of a paranoid type, with ideas of reference, fears of being poisoned or gassed, delusions of being spied upon, having one's telephone tapped or in other ways being persecuted and threatened with harm. A shared hallucination, either auditory or visual, is more unusual but is occastionally reported.

EXAMINATION OF THE PARENT AND CHILD:

1. On examination, an extremely close attachment between the partners sharing the psychosis can be noted.

2. The two partners often live in relative isolation, avoiding others, such as neighbors or extended family who might confront the psychosis.

3. When the delusional partners are separated, the delusional ideas tend to persist in the dominant partner and tend to weaken or disappear in the submissive partner.

4. Often, the submissive partner is characterized by immaturity, dependence, suggestibility, passivity and poor contact with reality.

5. Separation and individuation in the child who shares the psychosis is incomplete, and there is a sense of "fusion or symbiosis" of the delusional pair.

TREATMENT:

1. Hospitalization of both partners of the delusional pair should be considered.

2. The strength of the delusion in the child may decrease as separation of the pair is accomplished; however, further decompensation of either of the members may occur at the time of separation.

3. Outpatient treatment of the dominant partner, possibly including the use of psychoactive medication, should be considered.

4. Outpatient treatment of a long-term nature for the submissive partner should be provided with a plan of encouraging age-appropriate separation and individuation.

: :

DELIRIUM

GENERAL COMMENTS:

Delirium is defined as an <u>acute,</u> <u>reversible</u> mental state characterized by confusion and altered, fluctuating consciousness due to an alteration of cerebral metabolism. Delusions, illusions and/or hallucinations are frequently noted in this syndrome. There is often an associated emotional lability, typically appearing as anxiety and agitation. The changes in cerebral metabolism which lead to the cognitive dysfunction may be due to a variety of toxic, metabolic, infectious, postoperative, traumatic, vascular, neoplastic, febrile or degenerative conditions. Engel and Romano (1959) demonstrated that patients with delirium show a characteristic slowing of the EEG which is highly correlated with the level of consciousness, ability to attend and the performance of cognitive functions. Other authors (Adams and Victor, 1966) stress the increase in psychomotor and autonomic activity. Any change in the familiarity of the environment or a decrease in sensory input tends to make the signs and symptoms worse. Symptoms are typically more prominent at night.

Although delirium is thought to occur more commonly in adult patients, it must always be considered when evaluating an infant, child or adolescent who presents with an acute change in cognitive, psychomotor or autonomic activity, especially when this change is associated with a generalized slowing of the EEG. This syndrome varies greatly among patients and may fluctuate widely within a single patient.

HISTORY:

Delirium is a medical entity. Therefore, a careful medical history from the patient and his family is essential. However, it is important to assess the patient's premorbid personality and current life situation as these may lead to an accentuation or diminution of a particular symptom. It is also important to consider the developmental level that the patient has achieved in order to make an accurate evaluation of the cognitive changes.

EXAMINATION OF THE PATIENT:

1. Diagnostic alliance: An interview to foster a diagnostic alliance should precede the more formal mental status examination. This interview should focus on:

   a) Biographical data
   b) The child's reaction to the hospital experience

2. Diagnostic evaluation: The following data are best obtained by making several brief visits over a few hours or days, rather than by making a single extensive evaluation:

   a) Orientation (time, place, person)
   b) Memory (immediate, recent, past)
   c) Identification of familiar objects (key, watch, pencil)
   d) Level of consciousness (fluctuation)
   e) Serial 7s or 3s (subtracting 7 from 100 or 3 from 21 down to zero, observe for speed, accuracy, number and nature of errors, perseveration or loss of place, recourse to

concrete guides, such as finger counting)

   f) Number of digits which can be retained and repeated forward and/or backward
   g) Ability to deal with abstract concepts (interpretation of familiar proverbs)
   h) Level of activity and attention
   i) Affect (stability and appropriateness)
   j) Awareness and interpretation of internal and external sensory stimuli
   k) Complete general neurological evaluation

SIGNS AND SYMPTOMS:

1. Cognitive changes:

   a) Disorientation (time more frequent than person or place)
   b) Defects in retention and recall
   c) Mistakes in the identification of familiar objects
   d) Errors in serial 7s or 3s - perseveration, skipping, recourse to concrete guides
   e) Faulty digit retention or inconsistent responses
   f) Inability to interpret abstract concepts (proverbs)
   g) Decreased attention span or hypervigilance

2. Emotional changes:

   a) Labile or inappropriate affect
   b) Illusions, hallucinations (most frequently visual), delusions or stupor
   c) Fears of being abandoned, attacked, being bad or somatic preoccupations
   d) Excessive guilt (over loss of control), denial or depression
   e) Provocative or disruptive behavior
   f) Interference with medical procedures or treatments

3. Physiological changes:

   a) Slowing of the EEG
   b) Autonomic hyperactivity - sweating, tachycardia, hyperventilation
   c) Agitation and restlessness
   d) Changes in regular sleep patterns
   e) Urinary and fecal frequency or incontinence
   f) Fluctuating levels of consciousness

DIFFERENTIAL DIAGNOSIS:

1. All disorders affecting and altering brain tissue metabolism should be considered.

2. Nonorganic psychogenic states:

    a) Patients with mania or depression are rarely disoriented.

    b) Functional psychotic disorders are not associated with the same generalized cognitive defects. Psychotic hallucinations, as a result of a functional psychosis, are more often auditory than visual. Olfactory, gustatory and tactile hallucinations strongly favor a diagnosis of delirium. Psychogenic disorders do not show a characteristic slowing of the EEG.

    c) Amnesia and dissociative states of psychological origin are manifest by disorientation for place and person much more than for time.

    d) Ganser's syndrome (pseudostupidity) can be differentiated by the consistently incorrect but approximate responses of patients with this syndrome (one plus one equals three).

IMMEDIATE TREATMENT:

1. Diagnose and treat the underlying organic disorder responsible for the delirium.

2. Structure and maintain a simple environment.

3. Provide orientation cues - a night light, familiar pictures of family members, a favorite toy or transitional object and a calendar.

4. Have familiar persons, parents, relatives or foster-grandparents available to help the child test reality on a 24-hour basis, if possible.

5. For each shift, assign the same nurse until the delirium clears.

6. Limit visitors to a few familiar persons until the delirium begins to subside.

7. Modest doses of major tranquilizing agents (Thorazine, Hal-

dol) can be used for extreme agitation.

8. Benadryl can be used for sedation (see Chapter V, p. 142).

9. Avoid sensory deprivation or overstimulation.

10. Avoid restraints.

11. Avoid central nervous system depressants, especially bar-biturates, as they often have a paradoxical overstimulating effect.

FOLLOW-UP TREATMENT:

1. Long-term medical follow-up will be necessary for those cases of delirium which are secondary to an exacerbation of a chronic illness. Stabilizing the causitive factors will reduce the likelihood of future episodes of delirium.

2. Psychological problems accentuated by the changes in cerebral metabolism may need to be treated following recovery from the organic illness.

3. The persistence of disturbed memory, perception or visual motor performance may require special psycho-educational intervention.

: :

DEPRESSION

GENERAL COMMENTS AND DEFINITION:

Depression in childhood has had a controversial position. It may be seen in a "masked" form or recognized as a modified form of adult depression. Rie (1966) summarized his review of childhood depression by saying: "The familiar manifestations of adult nonpsychotic depression are virtually nonexistent in childhood," Glaser (1967) and Toolan (1962) wrote of "masked depression" and "depressive equivalents," respectively. They included delinquency, school phobias, sleep disturbances and psychosomatic problems. Spitz and Wolf (1946), in studies of anaclitically depressed infants, described retardation of growth and development as a depressive symptom. However, in the same infants he observed the weepiness, sadness, withdrawal, poor appetite and sleeping disturbances that characterize depression at any age.

When the following factors are elicited in a history, the evaluator should consider a childhood depression:

1. Recent or remote loss:

    a) Parents, by separation, divorce or death
    b) Siblings or other relatives
    c) Pets or other symbolic losses

2. Deprivation or abuse

3. Acute or chronic physical illness

EXAMINATION OF THE PARENTS:

Three important family patterns emerge from Poznanski and Zrull (1970):

1. High incidence of parental depression (both as antecedent to and concomitant with the child's depression)

2. Difficulties handling aggression and hostility

    a) Temper tantrums
    b) Severe disciplinary measures (whippings, spankings, punitive weaning and toilet training)
    c) Marital discord

3. Overt parental rejection

EXAMINATION OF THE CHILD:

1. Children mask their depressions, in part to defend themselves and in part because they feel no one else wants to be burdened with them. The sensitive observer should note his own sad feelings that the child elicits in him and reflect them to the child for confirmation. Simple empathy like, "It's tough when all those things happen to a kid," will elicit previously masked affect.

2. A child defended against the affect of sadness can frequently express it through fantasy displacement. He may not be sad but the people in his stories are. Nothing good ever happens, and themes of mistreatment, loss, abandonment, injury and death abound. The depressed child has no ambition and doesn't know what he wants to be when he grows up, whether he will marry or if he wants to have children.

3. Even if not overtly sad nor expressing depression in fantasy, the child may reveal his depression by such defenses as denial and reaction formation, etc.

4. Another way the child may reveal his/her depression is by aggression, acted out against others or turned against the self in somatization or self-destructive behavior.

5. In summary, if the evaluator thinks the child is sad, feels sad in the child's presence or is struck by the child's bravado or other behaviors, then depression probably exists.

SIGNS AND SYMPTOMS:

1. Looks sad, unhappy, depressed and cries

2. Withdrawal

3. Expresses feelings of being unloved or rejected

4. Insomnia or increased sleeping

5. Autoerotic activities

6. Negative self-image ("mean," "stupid," "punk kid")

7. Aggressive behavior:

   a) Short, explosive, angry outbursts
   b) Teasing and bullying peers or siblings
   c) Somatic complaints

DIFFERENTIAL DIAGNOSIS:

Depression is the major underlying condition in a variety of presenting complaints. Insofar as delinquency, somatic complaints and school performance problems are manifestations of depression, it is essential that the depression be discovered and directly treated. The task, therefore, in the differential diagnosis is to find depression when it is disguised as other problems.

IMMEDIATE TREATMENT:

If the degree or depth of the depression includes a suicidal component, the patient should be hospitalized according to the principles in the later section on suicide and attempted suicide (see

p. 118).

After the child's depression is diagnosed and his/her safety
ensured, the next task is to provide or establish a therapeutic
relationship.

FOLLOW-UP TREATMENT:

A therapeutic relationship is the keystone of treatment. As an
outgrowth of the therapeutic relationship and the continuing diagnostic assessment, individual, milieu, drug or family therapy may be indicated.

: :

THE DYING CHILD

GENERAL COMMENTS:

The diagnosis of a fatal illness in a family member presents a
crisis for each member of the family. Each member's reaction
will depend on (1) his/her cognitive understanding of the meaning of death; (2) her/her previous experiences with loss or
death, and the actual or fantasied connection of the previous
experience with the present experience; (3) the existing family
equilibrium; and (4) the nature and quality of the relationships
between each family member.

Maria Nagy (1948) studied the child's understanding of death as
it related to his/her age and cognitive level of development.
The following is a brief outline of her findings:

1. The child between three and five years of age denied death
    as a final event. The state of being dead was a temporary
    one: "more or less dead." Children in this age group be-
    lieved that dead people could hear but not talk or were hun-
    gry, asleep or breathing gently. The most important con-
    cept was that the dead person was not with them at the pres-
    ent time but would come back.

2. During the 5- to 9-year-old period, children interpreted
    death in anthropomorphic terms. Death was a person: "Only
    those die whom the death-man carries off - whoever can get
    away does not die." This particular view of death by chil-
    dren may have been heavily influenced by the culture of the
    period, especially as reflected in paintings of death as a
    person, skeleton or frightening figure.

3. By the time the child was ten, death was understood as a final and inevitable outcome of life. Quotes from children of this age included: "Death is like the withering of flowers," "the termination of life," "Death is something that no one can escape," "Everyone has to die once, but the soul lives on." By the age of 8, present-day children commonly understand biological death as final and inevitable.

HISTORY:

The following areas should be thoroughly evaluated:

1. The developmental level of the child (cognitive, social, affectual and psychosexual)

2. The child's previous adaptive capacity (ability to master separation anxiety and the habitual resources, responses and defenses mobilized in the face of losses)

3. The existing and prior nature of the parent-child relationship

4. The existing family equilibrium and the family resources and defenses used in prior stressful situations

5. The meaning of the fatal illness, hospitalizations and medical procedures to the child and his family in terms of present or prior events and their actual or fantasied connections

EXAMINATION OF THE PARENTS:

The following should be explored in the interview with the parents:

1. Parental fantasies concerning the etiology of the fatal illness

2. Parental level of anxiety, fear or guilt concerning the fatal illness

3. Impact of the fatal illness on the parental relationships, parent-child relationship and sibling relationships

4. Impact on the extended family

EXAMINATION OF THE CHILD:

During the examination of the child, the following should be evaluated:

1. The child's understanding, real or fantasied, of the reason for the fatal illness (see general comments, p. 66).

2. The child's level of anxiety, fear, guilt or regression concerning the fatal illness

3. The child's ability to use mastery, habitual resources and responses, and psychological coping mechanisms to avoid pathological regression

REACTIONS OF THE PARENTS:

The parental reactions are similar to those described in the later section on reactions to illness, hospitalization and surgery (see p. 88), but often become more intense when the diagnosis of a fatal illness is established and more painful when the child has a relapse and is readmitted to the hospital. The following stages are usually seen in approximately the order presented:

1. Surprise, denial, disbelief, hopes of a mistaken diagnosis

2. Fear, frustration, inability to carry on normal routines

3. Projection of guilt, anger, bitterness, resentment onto the hospital staff

4. Depression, guilt, self-recrimination about genetic factors or not having obtained medical help sooner. These reactions are often accompanied by somatic complaints.

5. Mourning the loss "of the child that was and the child that was to be"

6. Rivalry with nurses or physicians, feeling that the professional competence in handling their child is a threat to their own parental capacities

7. Rational inquiry and planning for new roles

8. Implementation of new roles

REACTIONS OF THE CHILD:

The child's reactions are also similar to those described in the section on reactions to illness, hospitalization and surgery (see p. 88), but some reactions may be exaggerated while others are less prominent because of the need for more extensive denial. Any one or more of the following reactions may be seen:

1. Malaise, discomfort, pain, irritability

2. Disturbances in sleep and appetite

3. Regression shown by the reappearance of behaviors seen at an earlier developmental level such as thumbsucking; return to bottle feeding; demanding, clinging, negativistic behavior; regression in speech, bowel or bladder control; heightened separation and stranger anxiety. This regression may be seen in children with any illness but is usually more severe in a child with a fatal illness.

4. Reemergence of primitive fears and feelings of helplessness or inadequacy which may be initially denied and be more prominent on readmissions

5. Depression, including wide mood swings, hypo- or hyperactive behavior

6. Increased stereotypic behavior of a compulsive or ritualized nature

7. Misinterpretation of the meaning of the fatal illness. Pain or painful procedures may be viewed as punishment for real or imaginary transgressions.

8. Physiological concomitants of anxiety, such as tachycardia, palpitation, hyperventilation or diarrhea

9. Conversion reactions (see section on hysteria, p. 84).

10. Dissociative reactions, amnesia or pseudo-delirious states

11. True delirium

12. Psychotic reactions which may be secondary to either the illness or to certain medications, such as adrenocorticotropic hormones

13. Concerns over changes in body image. Antimetabolites and radiation may cause loss of hair, and steroids may cause moon facies and truncal obesity.

14. Mourning the loss of previous levels of functioning

15. Accepting new roles and limitations, or denying the fatal illness and pushing beyond limits, or giving up and becoming a chronic invalid

DIFFERENTIAL DIAGNOSIS:

1. Consideration must be given to the fact that many of the symptoms noted previously may be within the "normal" response continuum to the stressful physical, psychological and social stimuli that accompany the change from health to illness.

2. Emphasis must always be centered on the illness and the effects of the medical procedures to avoid the mistake of ascribing changes in the medical condition to purely psychological causes.

3. If there is a biological or experiential predisposition, a fatal illness and repeated hospitalizations may precipitate more serious and long-lasting psychological disabilities.

IMMEDIATE TREATMENT:

1. First hospitalization:

   a) All acute medical treatment and definitive diagnostic procedures should be performed in a hospital setting by physicians who will ensure the accuracy of the diagnosis and institute the most effective medical and/or surgical treatment. As Richmond and Waesman (1955) point out, ". . . promptness and skill in diagnosis of the physical disorder may have far-reaching effects, psychologically, in management."

   b) Binger, et al. (1969) suggest that once a definitive diagnosis is established, the parents should be informed, and questions concerning etiology, heredity, therapy, ultimate prognosis, problems to be anticipated, sources of help, and current research efforts should be answered.

   c) No definitive answers should be given to the child without discussing them with the parents and then should be given to the child only with the parents' permission. Parents may want to answer the child's questions themselves, or they may want the physician to answer them.

d) A good technique for answering a child's question concerning his/her illness is to ask the child what he/she thinks the answer may be. Solnit and Green (1963) suggest that "generally, the child is expressing three fundamental concerns by his behavior, direct questions and questions expressed indirectly:

(1) Am I safe?
(2) Will there be a trusted person to keep me from feeling helpless, alone and to overcome pain?
(3) Will you make me feel all right?"

e) A child should also be reassured that he/she will not be left alone.

f) Anticipatory guidance can help the parents and the child progress through the stages of their reactions to the fatal illness without fixation or avoidance of any one stage.

g) Psychological complications related to the diagnosis of a fatal illness can often be prevented when trust and communication are established early among family members and among the parents, child and physician.

h) Misunderstandings and confusion about diagnostic implications, treatment plans and follow-up services can be greatly reduced by having one physician as the person who provides the parents and child with all the pertinent information.

i) Issues concerning hospitalization and planning for surgical procedures are discussed in the section on reactions to illness, hospitalization and surgery (see p. 88).

FOLLOW-UP TREATMENT:

1. Following the child's initial hospitalization, the child's parents will often develop an insatiable need to know everything about the total disease. Sources of information include other parents who have children with a similar illness, friends, relatives, books, journals, newspapers, TV and radio reports, and other nonauthoritative sources. Therefore, it is important that the child's physician be in charge and be available to give an informed and meaningful explanation of the course of the fatal illness, the treatment plan that is being implemented and the reasons for not trying other yet unestablished treatments.

2. Parent groups which involve the parents of children with similar fatal illnesses may facilitate the anticipatory grieving process. This is the process by which the parents cope with feelings of loss, sadness and helplessness that occur when a child they love is going to die. The fear of "going to pieces" when their child becomes terminally ill may be greatly alleviated by watching other parents go through such an experience.

3. When relapses occur, the parents are again faced with the inevitable progression of the fatal illness, and they should be helped to build support systems within both the nuclear and extended family. Religious, cultural and personal philosophical beliefs must all be considered, respected and strengthened.

4. During the terminal phase, parents may feel resignation, "wishing it was all over." They may feel guilt, anger and frustration over the hospital staff's failure to save their child. The staff must try to understand the parents' feelings. The staff's own feelings of helplessness must not cause them to become defensive and unavailable for talking with the parents.

5. At the time of death, the staff can share their sadness in a supportive way, helping the parents to express their feelings and to make the necessary final plans.

6. A return visit by the entire family to their doctor or the hospital can be extremely valuable to help assess the normal process of the grief work and to help them raise any questions that may have gone unanswered. As Gardner (1976) states in such a sensitive way: "Personal growth is inevitable in any life task which is accomplished with integrity and dignity, including the task of dying."

SIBLINGS:

Siblings of a child with a fatal illness will also be exposed to many of the stresses which their parents go through. Issues concerning their own fate; feelings of abandonment when their parents are at the hospital; heightened separation anxiety; guilt; anger; depression; regression; and concerns about what will happen to their brother or sister after death are just a few problems that must be considered. However, most siblings will look to their parents for the answers to these questions. Therefore, a family that maintains open and frequent communication can best serve the needs of all of its members.

: :

GILLES DE LA TOURETTE'S DISEASE
(MALADIE DES TICS)

GENERAL COMMENTS:

1. This condition is characterized by the following behaviors (Woodrow, 1974):

   a) Sudden involuntary movements (tics)

   b) Explosive involuntary utterances, including:

      (1) Inarticulate noises (coughs, barks, yelps, grunts)
      (2) Articulated obscenities (coprolalia)

   c) Imitative phenomena including:

      (1) Verbal imitation (echolalia)
      (2) Behavioral imitation (echopraxia)

2. For the establishment of the diagnosis, only tics and explosive involuntary utterances are necessary.

3. The prevalence is estimated to be between 0.25 and four cases per 100,000 population. It is suspected that there are many undiagnosed cases.

HISTORY:

1. The course of this illness is remarkably consistent.

2. The age of onset averages 7 years with a range of 2-18 years. Approximately 85% of the cases have an onset of illness before the age of 10.

3. The progression of symptoms is cephalo-caudal:

   a) The first symptoms are usually blinking, facial twitching or neck movements.

   b) Later, movements of the shoulders, upper extremities and chest occur.

   c) The lower extremities are last to be affected, if at all.

4. The movements are brief and impulsive.

5. There is no associated EEG abnormality.

6. Vocal tics appear months to years later.

   a) Vocalizations are first inarticulate sounds, such as barking, grunting, clearing of the throat, animal sounds or plosives.

   b) Finally, obscenities are explosively uttered in about 50% of the cases, usually "shit" and/or "fuck."

7. Echolalia (imitative speech) and echopraxia (imitative movements) occur in 20-25% of the cases.

8. The symptoms are increased with anxiety, stress and fatigue.

9. The symptoms are helped by decreasing anxiety, drowsiness or sleep, and fever.

10. The course is usually progressive with waxing and waning.

11. Neither functional or neurologic deterioration occurs; however, the chronicity and morbidity predispose to suicide (Bruun et al., 1976).

12. The cause is unknown.

INTERVIEW WITH THE PARENTS:

1. Parents commonly bring the child in at the request of school authorities or because the child has been ostracized because of his symptoms.

2. They often note a sudden onset of the vocal utterances for which there is no obvious precipitating factor.

3. When there is a precipitant, parental separation is the most common.

4. On questioning, the parents usually recall that there was a period of only mild tics before the onset of utterances.

5. Often, one of the parents may be rigid, demanding, controlling and punitive.

INTERVIEW WITH THE PATIENT:

1. The patient's symptoms are usually the worst at the beginning of the interview when stress is high, but as the patient gains some support and relaxes, the symptoms usually subside.

2. The symptoms can be coded according to the following scale (Bruun et al., 1976):

   a) Mild: Symptoms are infrequent and inconspicuous. The patient can control them in public with complete absence of symptoms for brief periods.

   b) Moderate: Symptoms are frequent and obvious. There is some ability to control them in public, but there are no asymptomatic periods.

   c) Marked: Symptoms are frequent, obvious and bizarre to some observers. There is some ability to control them in public, but there are no asymptomatic periods.

   d) Severe: Symptoms are frequent, obvious and bizarre. They cannot be controlled, and there are no asymptomatic periods.

3. Intelligence is normal.

4. Personalities fall into two types:

   a) Extroverted: Friendly, gregarious, humorous, practical joker

   b) Obsessive-compulsive: Obedient, well-behaved, perfectionistic and anxious with marked difficulty in the expression of anger

   c) The latter type is more common.

5. In some cases, the tics may serve to allow expression of hostile impulses.

DIFFERENTIAL DIAGNOSIS:

1. The most important differential is with tics of childhood. In a clinical survey of 15 children, Golden (1977) found that the average delay from onset of symptoms to correct diagnosis was 4 years. He noted that in contrast to transient childhood tics, the nature and character of the movements in Tourette's syndrome constantly change. He noted that the child who presents with blinking of both eyes of rather acute onset, should be followed closely. The diagnosis of Tourette's syndrome is suspected when there is progression to other tics of a changing pattern. If the patient then develops involuntary vocalization, the diagnosis is reasonably secure.

2. Sydenham's chorea can be differentiated by an increased sedimentation rate. Post-encephalitic disorders can be differentiated by spinal fluid examination. Huntington's chorea can be differentiated by the fact that only one percent develop in early childhood, and that there is a positive family history. Wilson's disease (hepatolenticular degeneration) can be differentiated by a Kayser-Fleischer ring, decreased serum uric acid and ceruloplasmin. The verbal utterances are usually not present in these disorders and their age of onset is usually later (Bruun and Shapiro, 1972).

ACUTE TREATMENT:

1. After the diagnosis is made, if the symptoms are not disabling to the patient or family, no treatment is indicated except for close follow-up. Because of the progressive nature of Tourette's syndrome, the family and patient should not be blandly reassured.

2. If the symptoms are disabling to the patient or family, a therapeutic trial with Haldol (haloperidol) is indicated, since many studies have now shown Tourette's syndrome to be unresponsive to, or to have at best, an equivocal response to behavior therapy, psychotherapy, minor tranquilizers, anticonvulsants, electroshock, lobotomy and hypnosis (Woodrow, 1974).

3. The majority of children will have a rapid initial response. All of Golden's (1977) patients (average age 10 years) responded to doses as low as 1.0 - 1.5 mg/day of haloperidol.

FOLLOW-UP TREATMENT:

1. Symptoms tend to recur, and if they are not a transient response to stress, the dose of Haldol can be increased.

2. The dose is titrated against clinical symptoms and the appearance of the side-effect of an extrapyramidal reaction. The family must be warned about the possibility of this reaction and can be given a supply of 25 mg Benadryl, one or two of which can be given to the patient if this occurs. If the symptoms are particularly severe or unresponsive to low doses of Haldol, the child can be hospitalized and the dose increased more rapidly. The pediatric dose range is between one and five mg Haldol (Golden, 1977). In adult patients, the dose ranges from 6 to 180 mg daily (Shapiro, et al., 1973).

3. Overall response to medication has been consistent in that from 75-90% of the patients have had good to marked improvement with medication.

4. Despite single case reports (Kelman, 1965), psychotherapy is not generally effective for symptom control but can be very useful in aiding the patient in making an adjustment to the social consequences of his disease.

5. If medication is stopped, symptoms usually return in two to seven days.

: :

GROUP HYSTERIA

GENERAL COMMENTS AND DEFINITION:

There have been occasions in which symptoms of an hysterical nature have occurred in groups of children. Any of the symptoms described in the later section on hysteria (see p. 84) can be seen, although symptoms such as fainting or "swooning" are probably the most common. Attacks of dancing mania have also been reported. Although such epidemics are rare in modern times, they are still occasionally seen (Schuler and Parenton, 1943; Caulfield, 1943).

HISTORY:

1. The usual history given is that of a sudden onset of symptoms such as fainting, uncontrolled weeping, uncontrolled

movement or overemotionality in a group of children who are in close social contact.

2. The person to develop symptoms first is likely to be a highly respected or admired leader of the group.

3. Hysterical symptoms in the leader of the group often set off similar attacks in other members of the group.

TREATMENT:

1. Identification of the leader of the group is the first step.

2. Often a low-key, calm and reasonable discussion of the symptoms along with explanations of the contágious nature of the symptoms and the nonorganic base of the symptoms will result in relief.

3. Separation of the leader from the remainder of the group may be necessary on a short- or long-term basis.

4. If anxiety over a real or threatened loss or other traumatic event seems to be prominent, brief crisis treatment is indicated.

5. To treat anxiety, an oral anxiolytic agent may be indicated (see Chapter V, p. 143).

: :

HYPERKINETIC SYNDROME

GENERAL COMMENTS:

The hyperactive or hyperkinetic child syndrome was first described hundreds of years ago. The earliest accurate clinical description of the hyperactive child syndrome was by a German physician, Heinrich Hoffmann, in 1845, in a poem entitled "Fidgety Phil." Other terms used to describe the syndrome include "brain damage syndrome," "minimal brain damage syndrome" and "minimal brain dysfunction." It should be noted that the term "hyperactive child" does not imply a diagnosis nor does it imply any specific etiology but described a collection of behavioral manifestations that appear together.

HISTORY FROM PARENTS:

History obtained from parents usually includes the cardinal features of (1) hyperactivity (2) distractibility (3) impulsivity

(4) excitability and (5) other symptoms.

1. Hyperactivity often begins at an early age. The children require less than the usual amount of sleep and have more than the usual amount of energy. They wear out their clothes and possessions much faster than other children in the family, talk a great deal and are unable to keep still or keep their hands to themselves. Even when not hyperactive, their activity is often more intrusive and inappropriate than that of other children.

2. Distractibility is often a symptom of the hyperactive syndrome. These children attend to extraneous stimuli and are unable to "screen out" common background auditory and visual stimuli. They daydream frequently and are unable to listen in a sustained way to parents or teachers. They are often unable to direct their attention to or attend to a task in a sustained way.

3. Impulsivity is a prominent feature. These children often use poor judgment and frequently place themselves in positions of danger. They blurt out answers impulsively without reflection and often talk rapidly in a driven way.

4. Excitability is frequently noted. Temper tantrums that are long and severe are frequent, and often the child cannot be consoled. Unprovoked fights with other children are common. The child has low frustration tolerance and tolerates large groups poorly. He/she is often difficult to manage around holiday times and is usually easily aroused or elated.

5. Other symptoms that are sometimes present in the hyperactive syndrome include anti-social behavior, cognitive and learning disabilities, depression, low self-esteem and lack of ambition.

DIFFERENTIAL DIAGNOSIS OF THE
HYPERACTIVE SYNDROME
(Schmitt, et al. , 1973; Werry, 1968):

1. Developmental hyperactivity represents approximately 42% of hyperactive children (Schmitt, et al. , 1973). Developmental hyperactivity is characterized by the following points:

    a) There is usually no history of past neurological injury.
    b) The neurological review of systems is negative.
    c) There is no history of mental deterioration.
    d) The neurological examination is within normal limits.

    e) There is no mental retardation.
    f) The onset is often at birth.
    g) Concomitant emotional problems are usually not present.
    h) A family history of hyperactivity, particularly in males, is common.

2. Neurological hyperactivity usually represents 15% of hyper-active children (Schmitt, et al., 1973). Included within this category are children with so-called "minimal brain dys-function," which is usually chronic and static, and a much smaller group of children with acute, progressive central nervous system degeneration. Children with "minimal brain dysfunction" can be differentiated from other children with hyperactivity by the following points:

    a) There is sometimes a history of past neurological injury. A low Apgar score at birth or a history of previous fetal wastage (stillbirths, spontaneous abortions) may be present.
    b) The neurological review of systems may be either positive or negative.
    c) Mental deterioration is usually not present.
    d) Neurological examination often shows "soft signs" which include:
        (1) Clumsiness
        (2) Confused laterality
        (3) Mixed dominance
        (4) Constructional apraxia
        (5) Difficulty with complicated movements, synkinesias
        (6) Jerky visual tracking
        (7) Mild hyperreflexes in the lower extremities
        (8) Speech difficulties
        (9) Difficulties with rapidly alternating movements.
    e) "Hard" neurological signs are rarely found.
    f) Mental retardation is usually not present.
    g) The age of onset is variable but may follow an identifiable CNS injury.
    h) Severe emotional problems may be absent or present.

3. Mental retardation can be a cause of hyperactivity and may be seen in approximately 6% of children referred because of hyperactivity (Schmitt, et al., 1973). Points that differen-tiate this kind of hyperactivity from others include:

    a) A history of past neurological injury may be positive or negative.
    b) A neurological review of systems is usually negative.
    c) Progressive mental deterioration is usually not present

and the amount of impairment is usually static.
d) A neurological examination may reveal both "hard" and "soft" neurological signs.
e) Mental retardation is always present.
f) The age of onset is variable.
g) Severe emotional problems are usually not present.

4. <u>Psychogenic hyperactivity</u> of either a severe or mild degree may be caused by the following conditions:

   a) Situational anxiety
   b) Parental overreaction to other types of behavior
   c) Maternal deprivation
   d) Severe neurosis
   e) Childhood psychosis

   Psychogenic hyperactivity probably accounts for about 37% of childhood hyperactivity (Schmitt, et al. , 1973). Psychogenic hyperactivity can be differentiated from the other types of hyperactivity by the following points:

   a) There is usually no history of past neurological injury.
   b) The neurological review of systems is usually negative.
   c) Mental deterioration is not present.
   d) Neurological examination is unremarkable.
   e) Mental retardation is usually not present.
   f) The age of onset is usually after the age of two.
   g) Severe emotional problems may be a cause or a result of the hyperactivity.

EXAMINATION OF THE CHILD AND PARENTS:

1. Evaluation should include a developmental history and a family history with special attention to the following points:

   a) Previous history of fetal wastage
   b) Perinatal events including maternal infection, high fever, prematurity, maternal addictions, seizures, neurological trauma, etc.
   c) History of symptoms, including age of onset
   d) Parental and sibling history of hyperactivity
   e) Parental history of sociopathy, learning problems and alcoholism

2. An office observation of the child and the parents together is useful (a) in defining the aspects of the child-parent interaction that contribute to the hyperactivity and (b) in noting parental management of the hyperactive child.

3. An electroencephalogram is usually noncontributory, unless there is a question of a seizure disorder or brain damage.

TREATMENT:

Fish (1971) has commented on the "one child, one drug" myth in the use of stimulants in the treatment of childhood hyperactivity. A combination of treatment modalities is always required in the treatment of hyperactive children.

1. Parental counseling:

   a) Parental counseling is especially useful in developmental hyperactivity but should also be used in neurological hyperactivity, psychogenic hyperactivity and hyperactivity resulting from mental retardation.

   b) Parental counseling directed toward relieving parents' guilt over their presumed role in causing the hyperactivity can be useful in developmental or neurological hyperactivity.

   c) Keeping a diary of events and episodes is often useful. In this diary, the A, B, Cs of the events can be recorded. The A, B, Cs are:

      (1) What are the Antecedents of the events?
      (2) What is the Behavior that is seen?
      (3) What are the Consequences that the parents offer to the child?

   d) Keeping a chart of target behaviors is also useful, and parents may wish to institute a reward system to help increase the frequency of desirable behaviors and decrease the frequency of undesirable behaviors.

   e) Individual child psychotherapy focused on the anxieties, concerns and family conflicts experineced by the child can be useful in conjunction with parental counseling.

2. Educational treatment:

   a) The teacher can be an important ally in the treatment of a hyperactive child. He/she is likely to be a more accurate and objective observer of the child's behavior than parents and can note the child's response or nonresponse to medication. He/she will often be able to assist in any system of rewards or management that is set up and extend the influence of the treatment program over a larger segment of the child's life (Farley and Blom, 1976).

   b) Teachers can be alert to any concurrent learning or cog-

nitive problems accompanying the hyperactivity and arrange appropriate remediation when needed.

c) It may be useful to suggest a classroom that is small, not
open, self-contained, predictable and structured.

d) A teacher should be sought who is clear in her expectations and instructions and consistent in offering consequences for the child's behavior.

e) Since hyperactivity tends to decrease with age, consideration may be given to retaining a child for an extra year
in a preschool program.

3. Pharmacological therapy: Stimulant medications can be of
immense help but should not be used as the initial treatment
modality. The use of medication by itself in treatment of
hyperactivity is not indicated. Medication should only be
used when combined with parent counseling, educational
treatment and at times child psychotherapy (see Chapter V
for medications and dosages, p. 141).

4. Unproven treatments: Unproven treatments for hyperactivity
include the following:

a) Megavitamin therapy
b) Orthomolecular therapy
c) Use of mineral or trace elements
d) Lithium carbonate
e) Caffeine
f) Antihistamines
g) Hypo-allergenic diets
h) Sugar-free diets
i) Additive- and salicylate-free diets
j) Patterning exercises
k) Visual training
l) Vestibular stimulation
m) Bio-feedback alpha wave conditioning

All the previously mentioned treatments are currently of unproven value, and some, such as lithium carbonate, have
considerable risk.

: :

HYSTERIA

GENERAL COMMENTS:

There is a great deal written about hysteria in adults, but less has been written about hysteria in children. Hysteria in adults was one of the earliest recognized psychiatric disorders. The word hysteria comes from the Greek word hysteron, meaning uterus. Hippocrates coined the word hysteria and felt that the disease was a result of a "wandering uterus." There has long been the implication that hysteria is in some way linked with repressed sexual desires or impulses. Hippocrates felt that hysteria was a convulsive disorder occurring only in women who were unfulfilled sexually, namely spinsters and widows. In 1853, Robert Carter stated: "Sexual passion is by far the most frequent and important of all immediate etiological a-gents." Freud (1896) felt that hysteria was a result of forbid-den or unacceptable sexual wishes that were unconscious and were expressed by way of symptom formation. Many have noted the unusual suggestibility of those who have hysteria. The inci-dence of hysterical symptoms in both children and adults is de-creasing (Veith, 1965). Hysteria is also said to be seen more frequently in areas of the country and in subcultures where sev-eral factors combine (Proctor, 1958, 1967). Among these fac-tors are the following:

1. Little functional anatomical knowledge

2. Authoritarian child-rearing patterns

3. Persistence and encouragement of magical thinking

4. Suppression of sexual and aggressive impulses, both in thought and deed

5. Stimulation of child's sexual wishes by parents

DEFINITION:

The characteristic clinical features of hysteria are:

1. A physical manifestation without a demonstrable anatomical explanation

2. A calm mental attitude called "la belle indifference"

3. Episodic mental states in which a limited but homogeneous group of functions occupies the field of consciousness, often

to the complete exclusion of the usual contents of consciousness, such as fugues, somnabulisms, dream-states, hypnotic states, etc.

There is a dissociation of the mental or bodily functions, and the dissociated function may operate in coexistence with normal consciousness, or it may operate to the exclusion of the other functions. Hysteria frequently includes four types of symptoms: motor, sensory, visceral and mental.

FAMILY AND CHILD HISTORY:

In the evaluation of the child and the family in the emergency room, the examiner should consider the following questions:

1. What might the unconscious meaning of the symptom be to the child?

2. What is the possible secondary gain of the symptom to the child?

3. What are parents doing either consciously or unconsciously to maintain and encourage the symptom?

4. Is the child or are the parents concerned about the symptom? Are they indifferent?

5. Is there an important figure in the child's life from whom he/she has learned the symptom?

An hysterical symptom should meet the following criteria:

1. The symptom should be a symbolic expression of an unconscious conflict between a forbidden wish or impulse and a fear of punishment.

2. The patient should show indifference to the symptom.

3. A large measure of secondary gain should be connected with the symptom.

4. The symptom should represent an unconscious identification with a characteristic of an important person in the patient's life.

SIGNS AND SYMPTOMS:

The distribution of these symptoms is rarely along expectable anatomic lines and is likely to vary from examination to examination.

1. Motor symptoms:

    a) Paralysis with or without contractures
    b) Tics
    c) Tremors
    d) Muscular weakness
    e) Astasia-Abasia

2. Sensory symptoms:

    a) Anesthesia
    b) Paresthesia
    c) Hyperesthesia
    d) Blindness
    e) Deafness
    f) Loss of gustatory sensation

3. Visceral Symptoms:

    a) Bulimia
    b) Anorexia
    c) Vomiting
    d) Respiratory tic
    e) Feeling of fullness
    f) Flatulence

4. Mental symptoms:

    a) Hysterical "fits" or "attacks"
    b) Trance-like or dream-like states
    c) Fugues
    d) Amnesias
    e) Somnambulisms
    f) Attacks of rage or impulsive behavior

DIFFERENTIAL DIAGNOSIS:

Hysteria should be carefully differentiated from a variety of organic illnesses by a thorough medical history and physical examination. Included in the differential diagnosis are the following:

1. Multiple sclerosis

2. Gilles de la Tourette's disease

3. Epilepsy

4. Drug intoxication or adverse reaction to drug administration, especially major tranquilizers

5. Brain tumors

6. Childhood psychosis

7. Degenerative neurological disorders

TREATMENT

1. Psychodynamic approaches: In this approach, the treatment
helps the child understand the symbolic meaning of the hysterical symptom or symptoms. The unconscious impulses
and wishes are brought to consciousness, and the unconscious expected punishment for those wishes is also understood. The secondary gain that accrues to the patient
from the symptoms is recognized, and the important identification figure, and the meaning of that figure to the child
are discussed. This approach is usually not used in the
emergency room setting and must take place over an extended period of time in an outpatient setting.

2. Behavior modification approaches: In these approaches, the
effort in treatment is directed toward understanding and
changing ways in which the hysterical symptom or symptoms
are rewarded either by the child's environment or by the
child himself. Antecedents to the symptom expression are
noted, and the environmental consequences offered following the expression of the symptom are carefully recorded.
Rewards for the symptom are removed, or other behavior
that is incompatible with the symptom is encouraged and
takes the place of the symptom.

This work may be initiated in the emergency room but will
probably need to be carried on over a several month period
in outpatient treatment.

3. Family approaches: In these approaches the child's
hysterical symptom or symptoms are seen as expressions of family conflict, tensions, communications patterns, forbidden impulses or punishment for those impulses.
The effort in treatment is directed toward discovering what
family conflict or impulse the child is expressing through
his/her hysterical symptom. The child is seen as being the
bearer and the expresser of the family conflicts. This work
is usually done in a series of family therapy meetings over
a several-month period. Special attention is paid to the function of the symptom in the psychic economy of the family
with the purpose of explaining how the symptom serves to

protect the family from conscious awareness of certain impulses and affects.

HYPNOSIS:

The use of hypnosis is the oldest method for the treatment of
hysterical symptoms and the one most used in the emergency
room. In this treatment, the patient, while in a hypnotic state,
is given a suggestion that the symptoms will be relieved. Several sessions or more are usually required. Since patients with
hysterical symptoms are suggestible, this is usually an effective treatment for symptom removal. With the use of hypnosis
for symptom removal, there has been concern that another
symptom may be substituted for the removed symptom, because the underlying conflict has not been resolved or dealt
with. This has not been a frequent occurrence. A variant of
this method is to use the hypnotic state to explore the unconscious conflict behind the hysterical symptoms.

MEDICATION:

Psychoactive medications, usually minor tranquilizers, have
been used with modest success in the treatment of hysterical
symptoms. The principal benefit from medication is usually
due to the placebo effect in a suggestible patient.

: :

REACTIONS TO ILLNESS,
HOSPITALIZATION AND SURGERY

GENERAL COMMENTS:

Acute or chronic illness, hospitalization and surgery are associated with a deviation from the normal state of adaptive
equilibrium which the child maintains when he is healthy. The
deviation, whether it is brief or long-term, occurs as a result
of the stressful physical, psychological and social stimuli that
accompany the change from health to illness. The child's genetic endowment, his developmental capacities, the supportive
nature of his family environment, his past experiences and his
psychological defenses play a major role in the determination
of the nature of the eventual outcome of these stressful stimuli.

It appears that children in the late infant and toddler developmental period, 8-10 months to 3-4 years, are the most vulnerable to the stressful stimuli associated with illness, hospitalization and surgery. Children in this group no longer feel totally
supported and protected by their parents, and their cognitive
development is not sufficient to allow them to understand what
is happening to them. Therefore, medical, surgical and nursing procedures are often poorly understood and/or misinter-
preted. Time concepts are also vague; a few hours may seem
like an eternity, and it is a period when sudden or prolonged

separation can be overwhelming and lead to panic or massive regression.

The young child who appears to be undisturbed by separation, or even happy, may be showing evidence of an unhealthy absence of separation anxiety. Likewise, the infant or young child who does not cry or fuss when a painful procedure is performed may have been repeatedly exposed to abusive painful experiences and, therefore, is no longer responding in a normal way.

Bergmann and Freud (1966) observe "that no greater gulf exists between the practical, factual, and realistic approach of most medical and nursing personnel on the pediatric wards and the unrealistic, affective, response of their patients - a gulf which may preclude cooperation and the building up of positive relationships, and causes as much exasperation on one side as it causes distress and unhappiness on the other." The task of achieving a relative inner balance is not an easy one for any child. It becomes immeasurably more difficult when the anxieties, frustrations and deprivations due to illness, hospitalization or surgery are added to it.

HISTORY:

The historical material should include a detailed assessment of the following:

1. The child's cognitive, social, affectual and psychosexual developmental level

2. The child's previous adaptive capacity. His/her ability to master separation anxiety and the habitual resources, responses and defenses mobilized in the face of previous danger

3. The existing and prior nature of the parent-child relationship

4. The existing family equilibrium, and the family resources and adaptive capacities used in prior stressful situations

5. The meaning of the illness, hospitalization or surgery to the child and his family in terms of present or prior events and their actual or fantasied connections

6. The nature of the illness: acute, chronic, infectious, traumatic, accidental, inherited, life-threatening or disfiguring

EXAMINATION OF THE PARENTS:

1. Parental fantasies concerning the etiology of the present illness, hospitalization or surgery

2. Parental level of anxiety, fear or guilt concerning the present illness, hospitalization or surgery

3. Impact of the illness, hospitalization or surgery on the parental relationship, parent-child relationship and sibling relationships

4. Impact on the extended family

EXAMINATION OF THE CHILD:

1. Child's understanding, real and fantasied, of the reason for the illness, hospitalization or surgery. This must take into consideration the child's level of cognitive development.

2. Child's level of anxiety, fear, guilt or regression concerning the present illness, hospitalization or surgery

3. Child's ability to use mastery, habitual resources and responses, and psychological defenses to avoid decompensation

REACTIONS OF THE PARENTS:

Parents' reactions to the child's illness will usually occur in the following sequence:

1. Denial and disbelief

2. Fear and frustration

3. Projection of guilt, anger and frustration onto the hospital staff

4. Depression, guilt and self-recrimination

5. Rivalry with nurses or physicians, feeling that the professional competence in handling their child is a threat to their own parental capacities

6. Rational inquiry and planning

REACTIONS OF THE CHILD:

1. Malaise, discomfort, pain, irritability

2. Disturbances in sleep and appetite

3. Regression (reappearance of behavior seen at an earlier developmental level: thumbsucking; return to bottle feeding; demanding; clinging; negativistic behavior; regression in

speech, bowel or bladder control; heightened separation and stranger anxiety)

4. Depression (wide mood swings, hypo- or hyperactive behavior)

5. Reemergence of primitive fears and feelings of helplessness or inadequacy

6. Increased stereotypic behavior of a compulsive or ritualized nature

7. Misinterpretation of the meaning of the illness, hospitalization or surgery (pain or painful procedures may be viewed as punishment for real or imaginary transgressions; fears of bodily mutilation may be related to treatment procedures, especially when these are related to the head, eyes or genital organs)

8. Physiological concomitants of anxiety (tachycardia, palpitation, hyperventilation or diarrhea)

9. Conversion reactions (see section on hysteria, p. 84).

10. Dissociative reactions, amnesia or pseudodelirious states

11. True delirium

12. Psychotic reactions (toxic or secondary to certain medications such as anticonvulsants or adrenocorticotropic hormones)

13. Changes in body image (especially with burns, trauma and certain medications)

14. Chronic invalidism

15. Evoked fears of loss of self-control and fantasies about genital manipulation or mutilation during anesthesia

DIFFERENTIAL DIAGNOSIS:

1. Consideration must be given to the fact that many of the symptoms noted previously may be within the "normal" response continuum to the stressful physical, psychological and social stimuli that accompany the change from health to illness.

2. Emphasis must always be centered on the illness and the effects of the medical and surgical procedures to avoid the mistake of ascribing changes in the medical or surgical condition to purely psychological causes.

3. If there is a biological or experiential predisposition, then illness, hospitalization or surgery may precipitate more serious and long-lasting psychological disabilities. These may include (a) situational or reactive disorders (b) psychoneurotic disorders (c) chronic personality disorders and (d) psychotic disorders (Prugh and Eckhardt, 1975).

IMMEDIATE TREATMENT:

1. Avoid hospitalization, if at all possible.

2. Try not to disturb familiar pre-hospital, home routines such as night lights, sleep rituals, dress preferences or other patterns of behavior.

3. Pre-hospital preparation for elective hospitalization:

    a) The parents should discuss hospitalization with the child's doctor. The parents may be given storybooks and booklets to help prepare their child (Wolinsky, 1971).

    b) The parents should then discuss the hospitalization with their child

    c) The parents and the child should then discuss the hospitalization with the doctor.

    d) The parents and their child may then want to visit the hospital.

    e) All attempts at preparation must take into account the fact that preparation done too early may lead to excessive anxiety, whereas, preparation done too late may not allow for the proper mobilization of defenses and other personal resources to master the anxiety.

4. In-hospital preparation:

    a) Clarify reality by giving the child as complete and honest a picture of the coming events as he/she can understand.

    b) Introduce the child to the pediatric staff of nurses, doctors, activity coordinators, teachers, foster grandparents, clerks, students and any consultants who will be intimately involved.

c) Introduce the child to the pediatric ward, including play areas, visiting areas, rooms, beds, TV areas, bathrooms, eating and sleeping schedules, ward policies and roommates.

d) Introduce the child to the hospital procedures. Real and toy equipment may be used to demonstrate procedures before they are performed (Adams, 1976). Puppet play and puppet "therapy" may help to prepare the child for surgery or other more extensive procedures (Cassell and Paul, 1967). The function of any special equipment that may be used, such as special beds, masks for anesthesia, traction, etc.) should be demonstrated and explained.

e) Introduce the child to the intensive care unit and its special equipment if the child is to spend time on this type of unit.

f) Preschool and early school age children should be given simple and brief explanations about procedures and surgery. Explanations should be repeated with opportunities for questions until misconceptions about the procedures or about parts of the body which may be affected are clarified. Simple drawings are often useful adjuncts to verbal discussions. Children may need reassurance that nothing else will be done or taken out at the time of surgery. Older children and adolescents may profit from more detailed anatomical discussions and drawings related to the upcoming procedures or surgery.

g) Preoperative medication, anesthesia induction and recovery states must be thoroughly explained. Preschool children should have a parent or a familiar nurse accompany them to the anesthesia room and be present during the induction and recovery period. Some children need reassurance that they will not awaken before the surgery is completed. Others may mistake the onset of unconsciousness as impending death and need to know that the "forced sleep" of anesthesia is temporary and will be followed by complete awakening and survival.

5. Visitations:

a) Schedules should be flexible and ideally allow for the parents to stay 24 hours. Pullman-type beds are convenient for overnight stays.

b) Parents should be encouraged to help with their child's care.

c) If parents cannot stay, a "foster grandparent" can be assigned to the younger patients whenever possible.

6. Communication:

a) Children have a natural need and wish to confide and share their feelings. For younger children, it is the parents' positive relationship to the hospital which enables them to place their confidence in the hospital staff and communicate freely without experiencing a conflict of loyalty.

b) Parents are often anxious and confused, and they need careful explanations, opportunities to ask repeated questions and to express their misconceptions. By avoiding critical and judgmental attitudes toward parents, the pediatric staff can help them minimize their guilt and self-recrimination. This will also help to maximize the development of a "therapeutic" alliance between the parents and the hospital.

c) The pre-hospital and inpatient hospital preparation helps the child to understand the hospital environment and the attendant medical and surgical procedures and helps provide an opportunity to anticipate the overall sequence of upcoming events. Through such preparation, the child is helped to master a situation which is almost universally unknown and would otherwise produce a great deal of uncertainty, fear and regression.

d) If the child is adequately prepared, open discussions between the child and the pediatric staff, geared to the child's level of cognitive development, combined with therapeutic puppetry, will often be sufficient to help the child master the majority of his reactions to illness, hospitalization and surgery.

7. Activities:

a) Activities should be encouraged within the boundaries of the necessary medical and surgical restrictions.

b) Activities discourage regression and dependency which

may increase and complicate immediate adjustment and subsequent personality development.

c) Activities help to transform the passive experience of hospitalization into a more active one and allow the child to become the active master instead of the helpless victim.

d) Activities should be organized and supervised by a specially trained activities coordinator.

e) Activities during the school year should include an educational program that is sanctioned by the school system to give credit for assignments missed due to short- or long-term hospitalization.

8. Special treatment:

a) Children who have a premorbid history of psychological problems or who develop psychological or management problems secondary to the onset of their illness, hospitalization or surgery may need to have consultation from a specialist in the mental health field.

b) A child psychiatrist, clinical child psychologist, psychiatric social worker or psychiatric liaison nurse can often help the pediatric staff understand the reasons for and the meaning of the particular psychological problem or behavior that is interfering with the optimal management of the medical or surgical condition. The mental health specialist can also work with the patient and his/her family to help them alleviate the anxiety and conflicts that may arise. Brief daily visits with the child and his/her family have been found to be more efficient than extended, less frequent sessions.

c) Special techniques, such as hypnosis, have been extremely valuable in helping children to tolerate painful and/or frightening procedures.

d) Group meetings each week, or sometimes more frequently, can help facilitate communication between patients and staff and among the patients themselves (Schowalter and Lord, 1970). These meetings provide a setting for the exchange of information about feelings of separation and isolation, ward policies, and surgical and medical procedures. Many of the fears and fantasies surrounding potentially painful procedures and the concerns about anesthesia and pre- and postoperative experiences can be shared and more completely understood. A supportive and educational approach is used with the major focus directed toward the reactions of the group members to their illness, hospitalization or surgery. For children who will have a more extensive hospital stay, group meetings may focus on deeper psychological issues. Again, puppetry, real and toy hospital equipment, and other techniques may help to initiate and facilitate the discussion among group members.

e) Behavior modification techniques have also been widely employed for specific treatment issues.

f) Medications can be used to reduce excessive anxiety, and they may facilitate the implementation of the other treatment methods that have been discussed.

FOLLOW-UP TREATMENT:

1. Explanations for mild regression or other predictable post-hospitalization behavior should be given in advance, so the parents and child can see this as characteristic of the normal reaction to illness, hospitalization or surgery and not as a personal failure.

2. Management of crucial phases in convalescence, such as diets, amount of activity, special routines, etc., should be worked out cooperatively with the parents and child before discharge.

3. Reintegration into the routine patterns of family life, school and peer relationships should occur as rapidly as the child's physical and psychological recovery will allow.

4. Supportive or intensive psychotherapeutic, rehabilitative or educational intervention may be necessary to manage the more serious complications of illness, hospitalization or surgery. Such programs should be formulated and implemented with the help of the pediatric staff, child psychiatrist, clinical psychologist, social worker, school teacher, recreational and occupational therapist, public health nurse and other professional persons in the hospital and community.

5. Fragmentation of services and poor patient compliance can be greatly reduced by having the physician in charge act as the coordinator of all follow-up routines and services.

: :

RUNAWAY CHILDREN

GENERAL COMMENTS:

1. Running away as a method of problem solving has been an American tradition from our forefathers who immigrated from an unfriendly Europe to the pioneers who moved West. Huck Finn, an American folk hero, was a runaway.

2. Today, runaways are supported by a society with an excess of money, leisure time and an emphasis on mobility.

3. Next to drug abuse, running away is the most common expression of disturbance among American youth. The incidence has been estimated to be 600,000 to 1,000,000 annually (Raphael and Wolf, 1974).

4. Most runaways come from suburban communities, more than half are girls, and the average age is 13 or 14.

TYPES OF RUNAWAYS (Family History):

1. According to Stierlin (1973), the families of runaways can be divided into three types: (a) binding (b) expelling and (c) a mixture of the previous two types which are referred to as delegated families.

2. Binding families are those that cannot allow the adolescent to separate emotionally or physically. These families create two types of runaways, the Abortive or the Lonely Schizoid, depending on the parents' investment in the child. In the Abortive runaway, the parents make it clear that the child must stay with the family, although their possessiveness makes for a conflictual relationship. The parents of a Lonely Schizoid keep their child close to the family while being cool and distant, though not overtly rejecting.

3. Expelling families are those that have been telling the adolescent to leave home for a long time, sometimes covertly, but often overtly, through the use of harsh physical punishment. This family style produces a child who runs away in stages, the Casual runaway.

4. The mixed binding and expelling families are ones in which the needs to bind the adolescent to the family and yet to expel him are intertwined. While the parents do not reject the

adolescent and want him to continue as a family member, they also want him to carry out certain of their own unconscious impulses; hence, the term "delegated families." Inasmuch as the parents' conscious and unconscious impulses tend to diverge, they produce intense emotional conflicts in the adolescent who is not sure which parental impulse he is able to carry out. A crisis occurs which results in the adolescent running away. Therefore, these adolescents are known as Crisis runaways.

EXAMINATION OF THE PARENTS:

1. Parents of Abortive runaways keep their children close to them by offering them a great deal of gratification for remaining dependent. The parental message is, "Have fun, but stay close to the family." These parents are then surprised that the child runs away, despite the opportunities for enjoyment offered within the family.

2. With the Lonely Schizoid runaway, the message to the child is, "If you run away, you're a bad person."

3. Parents of Casual runaways are notable in their ongoing neglect of, if not brutality to, their child:

   a) Sometimes this is hidden behind excessive protests of concern for the child.

   b) Whether the family is wealthy or not, the parents frequently shower the child with material goods and are likely to protest, "How could she do this to us? We've given her everything."

   c) On inquiring about discipline, one finds that physical means, such as spanking, hitting or slapping with straps or belts are a typical mode of punishment.

4. Parents of Crisis runaways give their children the message that they should run away on a mission that will satisfy the parents' unconscious needs and then return home.

   a) These journeys may satisfy id, ego or superego needs of the parents (Stierlin, 1973).

   b) The underlying parental conflict of the Crisis runaway often becomes apparent in the interview when otherwise tired or unconcerned parents suddenly show a great deal of feeling in their conversation or seem unusually interested in one small facet of their child''s behavior during the runaway episode:

(1) In the id-mission, the runaway serves to satisfy the parents own forbidden unconscious wishes for sexual or aggressive gratification.

(2) In the ego-mission, the child literally goes on a scouting expedition to experiment with life-styles and situations which the parents are unable to attempt themselves.

(3) In the super-ego mission, the child ensures bringing harm or punishment to himself in order to decrease parental guilt.

ACUTE TREATMENT OF PARENTS:

1. The child's exit leads to a sudden increase in parental affect, usually a mixture of guilt and anger. The parents' heightened affect and unconscious ambivalence over wanting or not wanting the child returned makes it difficult for the parents to act effectively. Therefore, the therapist should be active and directive in helping them locate the child as quickly as possible:

a) The parents should call the police to report the child as missing and also give instructions to bring the child home when he/she is found. Some police departments also recognize the parents' ambivalence by requiring that the parents file a report and a request for apprehension in person.

b) The parents should call the runaway's friends who often know, or at least have a good idea, where the runaway is staying. It is best to remind the parents that angry threats of reprisals toward the friends may delay getting information. The parents should also be told not to be discouraged if the child's closest friends are not helpful. They should instead inquire if there is anyone else who might be able to help and then diligently follow up these leads. More casual friends may be more able to comprehend that running away is not in the child's best interest and may be willing to transgress the adolescent ethic against "snitching."

c) Parents should call the local adolescent crisis center. Many larger cities now have centers just for runaways.

Though the existence of these centers is sometimes thought to encourage running away as a solution to problems, the centers have been helpful in offering an alternative to more serious delinquent behaviors that runaways often find necessary to engage in, in order to remain on the street (Raphael and Wolf, 1974).

2. The therapist should advise the parents that the adolescent often wants to be found and will probably "surface" at least once with a phone call. Remind the parents that angry accusations will again drive the adolescent away. On the other hand, guilt-laden promises of total forgiveness for returning home can only lead to later problems. The runaway will often want to bargain, and parents must be helped to convey to the adolescent that they indeed want him home but cannot promise complete compliance with all the demands.

EXAMINATION OF THE CHILD:

1. The Abortive runaway leaves precipitously, commonly in response to a friend's urging or support, since the Abortive runaway is too immature to try it on his/her own. With loss of the friend's support, he/she is soon returned home, often in a few hours, because his/her behavior passively demonstrates that he/she is "lost" and needs to be protected. He/she may, for example, stand in front of a police station.

2. The Lonely Schizoid runaway leaves precipitously, but this is often in response to some personal belief about his/her destiny, long held but suddenly acted upon. The Lonely Schizoid runaways are also soon returned, usually in a matter of days and often via some institution, such as the police department or a mental health center. These children are the most likely group to have left home because of an associated psychosis and might require hospitalization to treat the psychosis before being returned home. They may have tried to form some relationships while on the run, but these are usually only superficial and transient. These children report that during their runaway, they often loitered around some counter-culture "hangout," without actually interacting with anyone, or else simply walked around church yards or city parks.

3. The Casual runaway has often been moving away from the family for some time. There is a history of missed classes, followed by a suspension from school, which leads eventually to the child just not bothering to come back. No immediate precipitating factor for this group of runaways can be found.

They report that they were able to find other people like themselves with whom they formed easy but casual relationships. A transient life with casual sexual experiences and delinquent behavior is common. These runaways seldom return home of their own accord and are the ones most likely to be involved in serious criminal behavior.

4. The Crisis runaway leaves precipitously in response to his/her own and his/her parents' unconscious needs in the midst of a dependency-independency conflict. These runaways feel helpless, but also feel that they cannot express their feelings to their parents. They run to escape their feelings and express their anger at what they feel is parental suppression. These are the children who most often seem to be running toward something (unconscious solution to the family conflict), as well as away from something (helpless feelings). Their leaving seems to have a quality of a mission about it, and when this mission is completed, they return home, usually in a few weeks and sometimes on their own. The return of some may be precipitated by a recurring aspect of their behavior which eventually brings them to the attention of the authorities. Others may return by engaging in some obvious attention-provoking behavior which seems out of character, unless the examiner realizes that this behavior occurred after the runaways had completed their mission.

ACUTE TREATMENT OF FAMILY:

1. Try to meet with the family within 24 hours after the adolescent has returned home.

2. Inform the family at the outset that the therapist's purpose is to help them identify the problems that led to the runaway and help them find a solution that is acceptable to all of them. It is not to determine who is at fault.

3. Commonly, the adolescent is able to state what he/she wants, but needs to have his/her goals made more reasonable, for example, borrowing the family car on weekends versus having his/her own. The parents often have difficulty because they frequently couch their requests in negative terms, such as, "stop running away," "stop swearing," etc. The therapist should help the parents find positive things that they wish the adolescent would do, such as helping around the house or improving grades, which can lead to more rewarding interchanges between them.

4. The therapist's role during the acute treatment is very much that of a mediator.

5. Crises involving runaways can often be resolved in four to six, one-hour sessions.

FOLLOW-UP TREATMENT:

1. Long-term treatment is indicated when the family is unable to come to an agreement about what they want in four to six sessions. This usually indicates a chronic problem for the family as a whole and will usually require family therapy.

2. The Lonely Schizoid runaways are the ones most likely to have psychotic disorders which will require inpatient treatment. They are also the ones most likely to be the chronic runaways described by Jenkins (1971). These children often require a secure setting on a long-term basis since their conflicts cause them to run when stress, including the stress of treatment, occurs.

3. The Casual runaways also often need a residential setting to deal with their behavior. In many cases, their legal problems cause them to be placed in settings for delinquents.

4. Abortive and Crisis runaway problems can usually be treated in outpatient family therapy with an aim of uncovering and working through the unconscious conflicts of the family.

5. Whenever the therapist works with a family that has a runaway problem, it is wise to remember that family dynamics and the child's style will often dictate that the child will run sometime during the treatment. Realizing this may help the therapist in dealing with strong counter-transference feelings of anger and/or guilt when the child runs (Meeks, 1971).

: :

SCHOOL PHOBIA

HISTORY AND DEFINITION:

1. School phobia is often seen with a fairly abrupt onset and most commonly between the ages of five to ten (Waldfogel, et al. , 1957). The child expresses a very strong fear of attending school and a wish to remain at home.

2. It is often precipitated by an actual or threatened loss to the

child. This could be in the form of (a) death of a parent (b) sickness of a parent (c) change in a parent's work schedule and (d) move to a new neighborhood.

3. It is often seen in the context of a hostile-dependent mother-child relationship, and the child usually expresses the wish/fear that if he/she leaves the house something frightening will happen to himself/herself or his/her mother. Maternal ambivalence regarding separation is also a prominent part of the clinical picture (Kahn and Nursten, 1962).

4. School phobia is often seen in the context of previous severe separation problems, usually dating back to preschool or kindergarten.

5. Improvement of symptoms typically occurs after the parent has agreed to keep the child home from school for the day. Usually no signs or symptoms are seen during the weekend or on holidays.

SIGNS AND SYMPTOMS:

1. Fear of attending school

2. Fear of being separated from parents (usually mother) under any conditions

3. Fear of specific people at school or on the way to school

4. Somatic complaints without physical findings, including (Schmitt, 1971):

   a) Headache
   b) Nausea
   c) Abdominal pain
   d) Fever
   e) Chills
   f) Muscular aches and pains
   g) Diarrhea or constipation
   h) Fatigue, tiredness and sleepiness

DIFFERENTIAL DIAGNOSIS:

A careful history and physical examination should be conducted to rule out possible organic conditions. Physical examination and laboratory studies will be found within normal limits. Other conditions to be considered may include the following:

1. Actual rather than displaced fear of the school

2. Depression

3. Childhood psychosis

4. Invalidism secondary to chronic illness

5. School phobia may be a symptom of more serious, under-lying psychopathology, especially when seen in children who are in the preadolescent or adolescent age group.

TREATMENT:

1. Treatment should be directed toward an immediate return of the child to school and strict enforcement of the child's presence at school. This may entail getting school attendance authorities, teacher, school nurse, parents, the child and the mental health professional together for a meeting to go over the attendance plan.

2. Treatment of the family should focus on the relationship of the child to other important family members. The hostile-dependent nature of the relationship should be noted and underlying causes of this explored.

3. Individual psychotherapy may be recommended for the child. In this therapy, the child's underlying fantasies and wishes toward parents (fantasies of loss, rage, dependency) can be explored and more adaptive resolutions can be achieved.

4. Behavior modification of a type to desensitize the child to the feared situation at the school or the situation of separation may be effective (Miller, et al. , 1972).

5. Psychoactive medication may be used to decrease the child's anxiety while in the phobic situation. Minor tranquilizers may be used such as Valium (diazepam) 2 mg q. d. or b. i. d. or Benadryl (diphenhydramine hydrochloride) 25 mg q. d. or b. i. d. (For additional information, see Chapter V, p. 142).

FOLLOW-UP TREATMENT:

1. Continued liaison must be maintained among the physician, family and school.

2. Second episodes may be precipitated by additional stressful

situations.

3. The prognosis is favorable, and with treatment, 95% return to and remain in school (Coolidge, et al. , 1964).

4. Although successfully treated, some children may develop a constricted, phobic life-style as adolescents or young adults (Coolidge and Brodie, 1974). Therefore, continued follow-up is indicated.

: :

SEXUAL ABUSE OF CHILDREN: SEXUAL ASSAULT AND INCEST

DEFINITION:

1. Sexual assault is the most serious form of sexual abuse of children:

   a) In sexual assault the child's body is penetrated.

   b) Sexual assault, as used here, means intercourse, rape (intercourse without consent) and oral or anal intercourse.

   c) Incest, as used here, means sexual assault involving someone nearer in kinship than first cousins.

GENERAL COMMENTS:

1. In Jaffe's study of sexual abuse of children, 85% of the cases were accounted for by either exposure or indecent liberties, and 15% accounted for by intercourse, rape, sodomy and incest (Jaffe, et al. , 1975).

2. Incest has always been markedly underreported, due to the reluctance of family members either to report it or to press charges.

3. Convictions on charges of incest are rare.

4. When incest is reported, it usually results in a plea-bargained charge of indecent liberties or else the charge is dropped.

HISTORY:

1. The prepubertal girl often presents with genitourinary complaints, such as chronic urinary tract infection or vulvovaginitis.

2. It is often surprising to the emergency room physician that these conditions have gone untreated for a long period without an adequate explanation.

3. A chronic, untreated case of urinary tract infection, anal discharge or vulvovaginitis, especially one secondary to Neisseria gonococcus, should raise the physician's suspicion of incest.

4. In the adolescent, incest may present as conversion symptoms, masked depression, irritability, truancy, failing grades or as a suicidal gesture.

The following might be a typical history. The father, about 40 years old, is home alone with his oldest daughter and is drinking. Incest then occurs. The father threatens the girl with harm or family expulsion if she tells. The relationship continues for some time, often years, with the daughter a passive but seemingly willing participant, until some crisis occurs in the family. Sometimes this occurs when the father turns his attention to a younger daughter and the older daughter reports him, seemingly as a jilted paramour. More often, however, incest is reported because of an event extraneous to the incest. The mother denies any knowledge of the incest, though a detailed history suggests it would be impossible for her not to have known. There is no striking feature of the family except that they seem closely knit by today's standards.

EXAMINATION OF MOTHERS:

1. The mothers present as immature, passive-dependent women who seem capable of stoically enduring a great deal.

2. They often respond with little emotion to the report of the incest and deny any knowledge of it, although they have consciously or unconsciously fostered it by being sexually unavailable to their husbands and/or by taking a job that places the husband at home alone with the daughter.

3. These mothers tend to be chronically depressed and the victims of physical abuse by their husbands.

4. They are also noted to be dependent on their own mothers and to foster a maternal role in the daughters which includes a sexual role as father's surrogate wife. This arrangement allows the mother once again to feel cared for as a dependent child. Many of these women are not only holding a job but may be the only breadwinner in the family.

5. These previously mentioned situations may help to explain why less than one-third of these mothers take steps to change the situation even after the incest is discovered.

EXAMINATION OF FATHERS:

1. Many of the fathers will be unavailable for interview, having fled or been detained by the police.

2. If available, they will most likely refuse to participate in an interview.

3. If they are willing to participate in an interview, they are strong in their denial of participation in the act.

4. If the incestuous act is acknowledged, they usually rationalize their behavior by saying, "I would rather she learned it at home than out on the street" or "It is a father's duty."

5. These fathers usually come from poor and chaotic families (divorce, instability) where they had an emotionally deprived childhood.

6. The frequency of alcoholism and poor sexual adjustment is striking.

7. Despite popular views to the contrary, they are rarely psychotic.

8. Like the mother, if guilt is expressed, it is only over shame brought to the family and not because of any personal sense of wrongdoing.

EXAMINATION OF DAUGHTERS:

1. In the past, the girls have frequently been described as seductive and as playing at least a passively, willing role in the incestuous relationship. This assumption must be seriously questioned and seems especially invalid since most incest begins before puberty.

2. As the incestuous relationship has usually been going on for some time, the girl is not in an acutely agitated state at the time of the interview.

3. The interview should be done in a private area away from the noise and intrusions of the emergency room.

4. The interview should also be conducted with the patient separate from her parents.

5. With a preadolescent girl, the initial interview should include the mother, so that the girl can receive her mother's permission to talk about her feelings in a separate, individual interview.

6. Since incest arouses such strong feelings, some practice may be necessary before it is possible to say comfortably, "I think that maybe your father or brother touched your body or private parts, and that frightens you."

7. At the time of discovery, many of these girls are understanding, if not supportive, of their fathers and angry at their mothers, who have placed them in a conflicting maternal and spousal role.

8. The daughter's guilt seems related more to the discovery of the incestuous relationship and the family disruption than to her own complicity.

9. Participation is often not admitted, despite physical findings to the contrary. Nothing is to be gained by pressing the patient for this history at the time of the initial exam.

IMMEDIATE TREATMENT:

1. If this is the initial contact with the family, the physician informs the parents that he feels incest has occurred and describes what steps he will be taking.

2. In some states it is mandatory that incest be reported as child abuse.

3. The physician informs the parents that a report will be filed and that he has a duty to the child to see that incest does not continue.

4. This may require hospitalizing the patient until there is assurance that further incest will not take place.

5. A home visit by a public health nurse is necessary to ensure follow-up, as many of these families will move from their homes to avoid facing the ostracism of public exposure.

6. Supportive psychotherapy must be made available to the family.

FOLLOW-UP TREATMENT:

1. Despite some feeling that the younger child is less harmed by incest (Sloan and Karpinsky, 1952) and therefore deserves less stringent follow-up, it seems wise to follow a conservative approach and refer all victims of incest for psychotherapy on at least a trial basis.

2. There is much evidence that adolescent girls have several serious sequelae. Depression with sleep disturbances, weight loss, learning disorders and promiscuity, including prostitution, have been reported (Kaufman, et al. , 1954; Glaser, 1967).

3. Treatment of the father alone usually does not help.

4. In one British report, fathers were treated individually while the mothers were seen in a group (Rosen, 1964). It was felt that the group offered some solidarity and support for the individual mothers while undermining their stance of "I'm powerless to change this. "

5. Parents Anonymous and homemakers have been advocated but are of unproven efficacy as yet (Sarles, 1975).

6. One encouraging study indicates that family therapy offered at the time incest is discovered markedly reduces recidivism and allows the family to continue as a unit (Giarretto, 1976).

: :

SEXUAL ABUSE OF CHILDREN:
INDECENT EXPOSURE AND INDECENT LIBERTIES

GENERAL COMMENTS AND DEFINITION:

1. Indecent exposure is by far the most common form of childhood sexual abuse.

   a) Jaffe noted that of 300 cases reported in a large metropolitan county, almost half were for <u>indecent exposure</u> with a peak frequency during the vacation months of June, July and August (Jaffe, et al., 1975).

b) Most of the offenses occurred in the afternoon.

c) A typical history would be that of a girl playing at a schoolyard playground with friends. A man approaches who may have learned the girl's name by asking one of her playmates. He tells her that he has an important message from her mother and takes her away from her playmates. He then exposes himself. Often, he will have an erection and masturbate during the exposure. No attempt is made to pursue the victim as she runs away. She tells her parents, who notify the police. The man is apprehended and he has usually had previous offenses.

2. Indecent liberties is a legal term covering a wide variety of behavior but here is used to mean looking at, manipulating or kissing a child's genitals.

a) The victim is touched, but he/she is not physically harmed.

b) The child may complain that "somebody played funny with me" or "played with my private parts."

c) Jaffe indicated that nearly 40% of his cases fell into this category (Jaffe, et al., 1975).

EXAMINATION OF THE CHILD AND PARENTS:

1. The most important question to be answered is whether the victim knew the man.

2. Usually the child is quite willing to tell his/her parents if a stranger performed the act.

3. When the child is less willing to talk about who did it, a person known to the child is more likely to be involved. This has far more serious psychological implications.

4. The child is most often unharmed physically, and only a brief physical exam should be performed to confirm this.

5. The child may be upset over the events because of excessive concern shown by the parents.

IMMEDIATE TREATMENT:

1. Since the child may feel guilty because of the incident or because of the excessive concern shown by parents, he/she should be told that "some men who have an emotional problem do this to children. The best thing to do is run away. It's not your fault."

2. Interrogation of the child should be avoided.

3. This is an instance where the excessive feelings and the response of the parents may cause greater harm than the act itself. The parents should be told that there is presently no evidence that children are harmed by a single incident of exposure or indecent liberties.

FOLLOW-UP TREATMENT:

Brief treatment may be indicated if the child shows excess anxiety, withdrawal, regression or guilt.

: :

SEXUAL IDENTITY PROBLEMS:
FEMININITY IN BOYS

HISTORY:

1. Femininity is uncommon in boys, but they will not grow out of it without treatment. Tomboyishness is much more common in girls, but most will grow out of it. It is difficult to predict which girls will not outgrow it. However, tomboyishness is accepted much more by society, and, therefore, not seen as a problem.

2. Femininity in a young boy causes much more distress to the boy and his family (other boys refuse to play with him, tease him) than does tomboyishness to a girl.

3. The most common referral age is 7-10, but with increasing community awareness of the serious potential of this disorder, the age at referral decreases.

4. Sexual identity is felt to be established in the first four to five years of life.

5. In one study, all boys with this disorder began dressing in girls' clothes before the age of six (75% by age 4) (Green,

1974). The most frequent age of onset was between two and three.

6. Femininity is demonstrated in several areas:

   a) Women's clothing: High heeled shoes are the most fre-
      quently worn items. Bathrobes and large towels are used
      to improvise dresses. Costume jewelry may be borrowed
      or improvised with paper clips and string. Cosmetics or
      felt-tipped markers are used for make-up.

   b) Peer relations: Relationships to other boys are poor
      (80% relate better to girls, 67% are described as loners),
      and only 25% are described as "good mixers" or leaders
      by their mothers.

   c) Gender preference in fantasy games: Fifty percent play
      the role of the mother and another 25% play some female
      when playing "house." Their favorite characters are Cin-
      derella, Snow White, the wicked Witch of the West and
      Dorothy.

   d) Toy preference: The favorite toys are female dolls with
      many costume changes ("Barbie dolls"). The boys resist
      their parents' attempts to change this preference to mas-
      culine dolls (G. I. Joe). They avoid cars and trucks.

   e) Rough play: Over 75% of boys with a sexual identity prob-
      lem are seen as participating less in sports and rough
      play than the average boy.

7. A typical history would be the onset of cross dressing in female clothes at age three, drawing pictures that are female,
   and using female fantasy characters and mannerisms (swing-
   ing hips). They choose girls for playmates and say, when
   asked, that they want to be a girl.

8. Usually, an adult outside the family (school teacher or
   neighbor) brings the boy's behavior to the mother's attention.

9. Often parents have been given false reassurance that their
   child will grow out of it.

EXAMINATION OF THE PARENTS
(Stoller, 1968):

In the examination of the mothers, the following findings are
common:

1. She finds this male child unusually attractive and responsive to being held.

2. She has had enough time to devote much attention to this boy, because subsequent children were usually born much later; she has few other outside interests.

3. Many of the mother's colorful clothing and cosmetic accessories are available.

4. Early feminine behaviors are considered cute by the mother and supported by laughter, more attention, or by showing off the boy. Later, the mother may be neutral toward these behaviors.

5. She may continue to support his femininity by seeing his playing with girls as a sign of an upcoming "ladies man."

In the examination of the fathers, the following findings are common:

1. The father is much less significant in the boy's life than is the mother. The father has minimal interaction with the boy when present and is frequently absent.

2. He supports early play with feminine objects or does not object to such play.

3. The father finds that his son is not interested in father-son and/or rough and tumble play and thus feels rejected.

4. He then feels that his son is a mama's boy and rejects him.

5. He later feels he has failed and then denies this by saying it's only a phase.

EXAMINATION OF THE CHILD:

1. When asked, he says that he wants to be a girl, hopes to become a woman, prefers the feminine role, but knows he is a boy.

2. He recalls parents initially liking his dressing up in girls' clothes.

3. He has often heard of men who were changed into women (Christine Jorgenson, etc.).

4. He may have an erection when cross dressing.

5. He may say that he dislikes having a penis or an erection ("it tickles" or "it hurts").

6. He may say he wishes his penis would go away.

7. He often wishes to have babies.

8. He is often exceptionally attractive and pretty.

9. To him, the father's role is poorly defined and unattractive.

10. When asked to draw a person, he consistently draws a female figure.

11. Commonly, the only male TV character imitated is one who imitates a woman.

DIFFERENTIAL DIAGNOSIS:

1. In transvestism, the boy has no question about being a male and wants to remain a male. He alternates periods of masculinity with periods of feminine behavior in which cross dressing occurs, but during which he enjoys his penis. He would never sacrifice his penis to become a female.

2. No childhood transsexuals have yet been observed to grow up to be adult transsexuals, but they have similar wishes and fantasies.

3. Casual transvestite behavior is common in little boys, but it is usually episodic, is done out of curiosity and results in embarrassment when discovered. It usually diminishes greatly by school age.

IMMEDIATE TREATMENT:

1. Inform the parents that he won't grow out of it.

2. Find a male therapist. This is especially important in order to provide the child with a male identification figure and male companionship if the boy is less than 6 years old.

FOLLOW-UP TREATMENT:

1. The goal is to develop a relationship of trust between the boy and a male therapist.

2. Help teach the child that it is impossible to change his sex.

3. Stress to the child the advantages of participating in some activities enjoyed by other boys.

4. Teach the parents to stop rewarding cross sexual behavior and showing it off in pictures.

5. Help the mother separate from her child.

6. Teach parents to discourage such behavior with single scoldings, followed by isolating the boy in his room for brief periods without access to female clothing. ("If you continue to do sissy things, you won't have many friends and people will tease you.")

7. Involve him in masculine activities with little chance of his being hurt (kicking a ball, running, going for a walk around a building, drawing, reading, playing board games instead of very competitive sports, such as Little League).

8. Encourage nonaggressive male peers to come over and play.

9. Point out to the boy his girlish mannerisms (walking, sitting or feminine gestures with his hands).

10. Several therapy styles have been used:

    a) Individual sessions with the boy and his parents
    b) Group sessions with several boys
    c) Teaching parents to act as therapists at home for certain target behaviors

11. Since the number of reported cases is few, they have not yet been followed to generate a useful prognosis.

: :

SLEEP DISORDERS: NIGHT TERRORS

GENERAL COMMENTS:

Disorders of sleep vary from the rather benign conditions of restlessness, sleep talking (somniloquy), nightmares and insomnia, to the more serious problems of the narcoleptic tetrad (narcolepsy, cataplexy, hypnagogic and hypnapompic hallucinations, and sleep paralysis), sleepwalking (somnambulism) and night terrors (pavor nocturnus).

Although they may create some anxiety for children and their parents, the first six disorders mentioned are seldom serious enough to be considered emergencies. However, the seventh, night terrors, may precipitate a feeling of sufficient emotional distress in the parents to require prompt intervention.

DEFINITION AND INCIDENCE:

Night terrors, as described by Fisher and his co-workers (1973), consist of a sudden change from quiescent sleep, usually in the first third of the night, to an active state in which the child shows violent bodily activity and marked evidence of physiological activation. The incidence of night terrors is about 1 to 3 percent of all children between the ages of 5 and 13 years.

CHARACTERISTICS
(Keith, 1975):

1. EEG characteristics:

   a) There is an impaired or partial arousal from stage 4 sleep to an awake (alpha) pattern.

   b) Seventy percent of night terrors occur in the first non-REM period of the night (15-30 minutes after the onset of sleep).

2. Physiological characteristics:

   a) There is a rapid increase in pulse rate, usually over 108 (often to 160-170 in 15 to 30 seconds).

   b) Rapid breathing occurs with a tremendous increase in the amplitude of respiration.

   c) There may be periods of apnea.

   d) There is an intense autonomic activation (sweating, mydriasis, etc.).

3. Motility changes:

   a) Excessive activity, such as thrashing about, sitting up and striking out occurs. Muscle tone is increased.

   b) Somnambulism may occur.

4. Verbalization patterns:

   a) Verbalizations are almost always present at the onset of night terrors.

   b) They usually include gasps, moans, groans, curses and occasionally blood-curdling, piercing screams.

5. Mental content:

   a) There is a single feeling, image, memory or thought of being overwhelmed.

   b) Elaborate dreams may occur in 10% of night terrors and these have a violent, aggressive, terrifying content.

6. Mental content, if awakened (the child usually cannot be awakened):

   a) The child appears confused, disoriented and unresponsive to the environment.

   b) Automatic, repetitive behaviors are observed, and the child is hard to calm.

   c) The child is relatively nonreactive to external stimuli.

   d) A retrograde amnesia occurs for almost all details of the event.

7. The duration of a night terror is usually one to twenty minutes.

DIFFERENTIAL DIAGNOSIS:

1. Nightmares (REM anxiety dreams):

   a) Nightmares occur during REM sleep and do not follow any particular time pattern.

   b) There is a gradual increase in pulse rate, usually into the 90s but little other autonomic activity takes place.

   c) There are fewer movements with no somnambulism. Muscle tone is decreased.

   d) Verbalizations may be present but are subdued.

   e) The mental content of nightmares is elaborate, vivid and of longer duration than night terrors.

 f) The child usually returns to lucid consciousness quickly. He is easily calmed and often has a clear memory for many details of the event.

 g) Nightmares may be much longer in duration than night terrors.

2. Delirium: Delirium secondary to drug intoxication or organic disorders is discussed in the section on delirium (see p. 59).

TREATMENT:
(Keith, 1975):

1. Night terrors based upon normal developmental conflicts are generally of mild to moderate intensity and frequency and usually last only a few months. Soon after their onset, there is a decrease in frequency, and unless a clear source of excessive conflict can be identified, no treatment is recommended.

2. Night terrors beginning after a traumatic event often require psychotherapeutic intervention.

3. Serious psychopathology is suggested when the night terrors are frequent (at least three to four times a week over a period of months), and this frequency does not decrease. In these cases, a psychological evaluation of the child and his parents is indicated. Psychotherapy and adjunctive drug treatment may be recommended.

4. Drug treatment has included a trial of Valium (diazepam) at bedtime.

: :

SUICIDE AND ATTEMPTED SUICIDE

GENERAL COMMENTS:

1. Suicidal behavior and ideation are the commonest psychiatric emergencies in childhood and adolescence. They must always be taken seriously.

2. Suicide is more common above age 12, and in a study by Shaffer (1974) no completed suicides were reported in children under 12 years of age.

3. Girls attempt suicide more often than boys but the ratio of completed suicides for boys to girls was 2.3 to 1 (Shaffer, 1974).

4. There is no apparent seasonal variation.

5. The suicide rate in adolescents has been increasing rapidly in the last few years (Conger, 1977).

6. The methods of completed suicides in rank of order of frequency are (Shaffer, 1974):

   a) Carbon monoxide gas
   b) Hanging
   c) Drug overdose
   d) Firearms
   e) Suffocation with plastic bag
   f) Electrocution
   g) Drowning
   h) Decapitation

7. The reasons for completed suicide, according to notes left by the deceased, in rank order of frequency are:

   a) Recently getting into trouble
   b) Rejection by boyfriend or girlfriend
   c) Fear of peer
   d) Parents' behavior
   e) Feeling of depression
   f) "A way out"

8. Of completed suicides, 14 of 30 (46%) had previously attempted suicide and 8 (27%) within 24 hours of their death.

9. Ten percent of parents of children who completed suicide have also committed suicide.

HISTORY:

1. In 76% of the children reported by Morrison, the event that precipitated the suicide threat or attempt was a loss or separation of a parent or parent figure, or the anniversary of such a loss (Morrison and Collier, 1969).

2. Long-standing problems in the family and/or child are almost always present.

3. Conscious and/or unconscious chronic rejection of the child

by his parents is commonly seen.

4. The previously mentioned conditions for a suicide attempt can exist for a long time or build up gradually, and the suicide attempt can be precipitated by:

   a) One more argument with parents
   b) An argument with or rejection by a boyfriend or girl-friend, especially when this relationship supplies love and support
   c) The school or another source planning to tell the parents something negative about the child

SIGNS AND SYMPTOMS:

1. Antisocial behavior, such as the following, may be seen:

   a) Bullying and fighting
   b) Stealing
   c) Truancy
   d) Running away

Comment: One should be cautious with patients who turn aggression outward, for it may represent an ineffective defense against a severe depression which may lead to suicide (Macdonald, 1967).

2. Emotional and affective symptoms, such as the following, may be seen:

   a) Depressed mood and fearfulness
   b) Hypochondriasis
   c) Excessive fears
   d) School refusal
   e) Self-denigration
   f) Feeling of worthlessness
   g) Hopelessness
   h) Feeling bad

3. Mattsson, et al. (1969) give the following typology of suicide:

   a) Loss of love object, followed by acute or prolonged grief
   b) "The Bad Me," markedly self-deprecating patient
   c) The "final cry for help" directed beyond the family
   d) The revengeful, angry teenager
   e) Psychotic adolescents
   f) Suicidal game

EXAMINATION OF THE CHILD:

1. Try to make a prompt alliance with the patient. The interviewer should not be seen as an agent of society or the family. This may help the patient reveal concerns and worries that he/she has not shared with others because of lack of trust. This is especially important with patients who present themselves as antisocial or aggressive. This interviewer-patient alliance can be accomplished by:

   a) Showing sincere interest in the patient and listening in a careful manner for both latent and manifest content
   b) Seeing the patient before the family "to get his/her side of the story" or asking the patient's permission to see the family first

2. Note the patient's mood and affect and observe the congruency of these with the content of his/her thought.

3. Ask about recent and remote losses and separations from important figures.

4. Ask directly about suicidal thoughts and plans, the duration of these thoughts and the seriousness of the intent.

5. Ask about feelings of the patient regarding the worthfulness of life.

6. Ask about the patient's feelings of self-worth.

EXAMINATION OF PARENTS AND/OR
SIGNIFICANT OTHERS:

1. It is most important to assess their attitude toward the patient and their response to his/her attempted suicide.

2. Continued suicidal risk is associated with the following responses:

   a) An attitude of indifference or lack of concern (parents fail to come to the emergency room)
   b) A punitive or denigrative attitude ("You can't do anything right")
   c) Minimization of the earnestness of the attempt ("I don't believe you really were trying to do it. You're just trying to get something from me.")

3. The degree of family stability and the amount, trends and

quality of family problems should be evaluated. The multi-problem family is less likely to have resources to help a suicidal child.

4. Inquire about the incidence of suicides, suicide attempts and serious depressions in these families.

IMMEDIATE TREATMENT:

1. The immediate treatment of any suicide attempt is to use medical lifesaving methods. Only when the patient is out of danger from the attempt are the psychiatric evaluation and prevention of another attempt initiated.

2. Hospitalization for safety has to be considered on the basis of:

   a) Degree of change in patient's wish to live
   b) Degree of change in the family system
   c) Degree of lethality of the attempt. The interviewer can assess lethality by considering:
      (1) The dangerousness and the child's knowledge of the dangerousness of the method chosen
      (2) The patient's efforts (conscious and unconscious) to be discovered before completion of the suicide by using letters, notes, telephone or direct verbal communication
      (3) The degree of impairment of judgment by psychosis or during intoxication
      (4) Accessibility of help

3. The factors just mentioned are only a guide. The decision to hospitalize is a difficult, critical judgment. The evaluator should use the maxim, "when in doubt, hospitalize."

4. A range of possible treatments following immediate treatment includes:

   a) Family therapy
   b) Individual child psychotherapy
   c) Residential treatment
   d) Foster home placement
   e) Psychoactive medication

: :

UNMARRIED PREGNANCY

GENERAL COMMENTS:

1. In 1970, 17% of all live births in the United States were to women 15-19 years of age, and nearly 30% of these were out of wedlock (Zelnick and Kantner, 1974).

2. Teenage pregnancies occur frequently throughout all social classes. However, they are most frequent among girls of lower socioeconomic status.

3. Konopka (1976) came to the following conclusions in open-ended interviews with over 1000 girls, 12-18 years old, throughout the United States:

   a) Unmarried pregnancy was a subject the girls thought about a great deal; it was definitely not a hidden or unimportant subject.

   b) The girls did not see simple solutions. Suicide or destruction of the child after birth was hardly ever considered. Only a small number felt that they would get married just to give the child a father and a name.

   c) Most girls wanted to keep their babies.

   d) The next largest group would give up the baby for adoption.

   e) Abortion was openly discussed. Almost half were against it. A quarter were for it and felt it preferable to bearing an unwanted child. Another quarter were ambivalent or considered it an individual matter. Most girls, even those against abortion in general, supported it when rape was involved.

LEGAL ISSUES:

1. In 1973, the Supreme Court ruled that a woman's right of privacy encompasses the decision to terminate a pregnancy. Accordingly, no laws may prohibit the taking of human fetal life in the approximate first six months of its existence. Abortions may be regulated by law during the fourth to the sixth months, but only to protect the woman's health. Laws may prohibit abortions after the fetus becomes viable, during the approximate final three months of uterine life.

2. In 1976, the Fifth U. S. Circuit Court of Appeals ruled that since the state had no right to interfere with a woman's right of privacy in the first trimester of pregnancy, nor before the fetus becomes viable, the state could not delegate this authority to husbands and parents. Therefore, parents cannot look to the state to prosecute a physician who performs an abortion against their wishes.

3. Common law has held that the consent of parent or guardian was necessary before medical treatment could be given to a minor. A new exception is the minor who is sufficiently intelligent and mature to understand the nature and consequences of a treatment which is for his/her benefit. This is referred to as the "mature minor doctrine" (Paul, et al., 1976).

HISTORY:

1. Teenage pregnancies are complex, including social, family and individual factors (Meeks, 1971). At least one researcher found that there was little difference psychologically or behaviorally in two groups of sexually active young women, one group of which had just had an abortion and another group which had never been pregnant. He concluded that chance plays a part in at least some of these pregnancies (Miller, 1976).

2. Semmens and Lamers (1968) described three categories of unmarried pregnancy arranged according to the amount of conscious participation by the girl:

   a) The intentional pregnancy, conceived in order to escape or force a change in an unhappy family life or as a hostile attack on the parents or the family name

   b) The accidental pregnancy, occurring in girls with a variety of unconscious motives ranging from those with dependency problems with their mothers in combination with absent fathers to those playing an unconscious role as the family scapegoat

   c) The unknowing pregnancy, occuring in girls who by ignorance or mental retardation do not know how to take contraceptive measures

3. For whatever reason, of sexually active female adolescents aged 15-19, less than 50% had used any form of contraceptive in their most recent intercourse, and only 20% said they

always used some form of contraception (Kantner and Zel-nick, 1973).

4. Aug and Bright (1970) disagreed with the generalization that unmarried pregnancy is by itself evidence of psychopathology. In their study of four groups of pregnant adolescent women, they found evidence of disturbed interpersonal relationships in both married and unmarried groups, and good interpersonal relationships in both married and unmarried groups.

Group I consisted of married girls with good interpersonal relationships. They had been raised in a stable family and learned good mothering behaviors by assisting their own mothers in the care of younger siblings. They gave the most comprehensive and favorable descriptions of their husbands, who held steady jobs and were without prison records.

Group II consisted of unmarried adolescents who had good interpersonal relationships in an extended family of origin. These families often included sisters who had also had an unmarried pregnancy. The mothering role was shared by all the postpubertal females in the family and gave the girls good mothering experiences. There was no interest in marriage to the putative father, and he was largely seen as unimportant. All of these girls kept their babies.

Group III consisted of married and unmarried girls who had disturbed interpersonal relationships and included runaways. These girls had been deprived in their family relationships, often from birth. Parents were often verbally and physically abusive toward each other and the children. This, coupled with the fact that the girls were often farmed out to relatives, resulted in their lack of positive mothering experiences. The putative fathers in this group often had histories of alcoholism and antisocial behavior. The husbands were often verbally and physically abusive.

Group IV consisted of girls who were married when they were between four and seven months pregnant and who had marked disturbances in interpersonal relationships. Their families of origin were unstable and splintered with parent figures seldom present for periods during the girl's early years; therefore, there was no opportunity for positive mothering experiences. Indeed, all of these girls were themselves illegitimate. The husbands, like those in the previous group, had histories of alcoholism and sociopathy.

EXAMINATION OF THE ADOLESCENT
(and Acute Treatment):

1. If an angry confrontation with the parents around the announcement of the girl's pregnancy has just occurred, allow the girl to ventilate her feelings of anger, guilt and rejection.

2. If she has not yet told her parents of her pregnancy, encourage her to do so as soon as possible and offer to be present when she tells them.

3. Explore with the girl her feelings about the pregnancy.

4. If barriers to informed consent can be ruled out functional or organic psychosis or such serious mental retardation as to deny competency), the girl can be informed that the decision to bring this fetus to term belongs to her.

5. Agree, nonetheless, to help her explore the various possibilities open to her, such as bringing the fetus to term, remaining unmarried and keeping the baby, placing the baby for adoption, having an abortion or getting married.

6. Try to determine if the motivation for the pregnancy falls into one of the groups with disturbed relationships discussed earlier, in order to make more specific recommendations for psychotherapy.

EXAMINATION OF THE PARENTS:

1. Allow the parents to express their feelings, especially anger, guilt and their wish to reject the adolescent.

2. Explain to the parents the various possibilities open to the adolescent, as well as any advantages or disadvantages about particular choices of which they may not be informed. Some studies show depression following abortion and a high rate of divorce in teenage marriages.

3. Try to elicit the parents' general support of their daughter, while allowing them appropriate feelings about this specific situation.

4. Remind them gently that their daughter has the ultimate responsibility for this pregnancy.

5. If, in exploring the parents' feelings, any evidence of paren-

tal psychopathology (for example, scapegoating) is detected, it will be necessary to assist the parents in seeking help for their problems. This is best done through a second therapist since the primary alliance of the first therapist needs to be with the adolescent.

FOLLOW-UP TREATMENT:

1. Minors who can give informed consent can consent to contraception, abortion and other pregnancy-related treatment, despite the fact that there is no specific affirmative statute in any state. In many, if not most states, teenagers who have the capacity to give informed consent may consent to all sex-related medical care (Paul, et al. , 1976).

2. A comprehensive approach involving cooperation and including obstetrical care, social casework planning and psychiatric counseling is best.

3. Remember that the therapist may have to go over many of the explanations originally given to the parents and adolescent since first discussions of such loaded issues as sexuality are frequently forgotten.

4. If serious but not disabling individual or family psychopathology has been discovered, this will have to be worked on concomitantly while discussing the resolution of the pregnancy. Frequently, successful treatment of such conditions will take longer than the duration of this pregnancy, but hopefully the therapist might prevent future pregnancies as solutions to conscious or unconscious conflicts.

5. The therapist's own values in this area eventually become obvious. It is best not to put the weight of these on the patient early in treatment, but rather to share them as they come up over some particular issue. Even so, it is important to differentiate those views which have some support in facts from those that are simple beliefs (Meeks, 1971).

: :

THE VIOLENT OR AGGRESSIVE
CHILD OR ADOLESCENT

GENERAL COMMENTS:

1. These comments concentrate on studies of dangerously aggressive children who are likely to constitute the most seri-

ous problem in the emergency room. However, the family dynamics and the child's general characteristics also apply to children with less severely aggressive behaviors.

2. Theoretical views of aggression vary:

   a) Freud, at first, felt that aggression was a derivative of Thanatos, a basic death wish, but later modified his view, identifying aggression as a basic drive in itself (Freud, 1920).

   b) Later theorists proposed that aggression was an innate tendency which needed to be socialized by a nurturing relationship in order to be channeled into useful and helpful directions (Hartman, et al., 1949).

   c) Lorenz (1966) proposed from his animal studies that aggression was a drive, the basic functions of which were to distribute a species over the available biological environment, protect the young and select strong species members through rival fighting.

   d) Bandura and Walters (1959) proposed that adolescent aggression occurs as a learned response to specific environmental stimuli.

3. There is general agreement that the frequency of crime by youths is increasing. Currently, from 10-12% of all adolescents and 20-22% of all male adolescents will appear in juvenile court before age 18.

4. Formerly, the ratio of boys to girls involved in serious acts of aggression was four or five to one. Since the late 1960's, however, crimes by girls have increased at a two- or threefold rate over the boys, so that the ratio is now about 3.5 to 1 (Conger, 1977). Many authors have commented that the increased aggressivity by girls is due, at least in part, to changes in societal attitudes that promote more assertiveness in females.

HISTORY:

1. In a factor analytic study of 500 child guidance clinic cases, Jenkins (1969) found that the group he described as "unsocialized aggressive reaction" was most prone to violent behavior. He found the family problems manifested in the following ways:

a) Children were unwanted; thus, the unsocialized aggressive child was likely to have few siblings or to be an only child.

b) Marriages were unstable, so that the child was likely to have a stepparent.

c) The mother was likely to be immature.

d) Parents were unable to agree with or support each other in disciplining the child.

e) Despite rejecting the child, these parents were likely to be somewhat overprotective and so try to shield the child from the consequences of his/her behavior.

f) Punishment, therefore, tended to be inconsistent. Severity was based on how the parent was feeling at the moment, or severe punishment was alternated with bribery.

g) Persistent enuresis was a common problem.

2. In a study of 9 youths (8 boys, 1 girl), all of whom had commited homicide, King (1975) noted several factors:

a) Brutal fights between the parents were typical.

b) All the children were subject to beatings, and the homicidal youth was the one most often singled out.

c) The children were inconsistently and ineffectively disciplined.

d) Episodic desertions took place, usually by the father who frequently left when a crisis occurred.

e) Problem drinking by one or both parents led to physical violence.

f) Many of the youths thought their mothers were afraid of them.

g) Most homes were intact at the time of the homicide.

3. Eron and his co-workers (1974) in a 10-year longitudinal study found that:

a) Parental punishment for aggression at home and rejection

by the parents when the child was 8, related to aggression at that age but did not predict how aggressive the child would be at age 19.

b) Children who had aggressive parental and television models at age 8, and who showed little guilt or rarely confessed to wrongdoings, were aggressive at ages 8 and 19.

c) The higher the social class, the more aggressive the female subjects; the more ambitious the father, the more aggressive the male subjects at age 19.

d) Ethnicity was not a good predictor of aggressivity for boys; I. Q. was not a good predictor of aggressivity for girls.

e) Low identification with both parents was the most accurate predictor of high aggression, whatever the subject's sex.

f) TV violence preferred at age 8 is one of the best predictors of aggression at age 19 for boys, but for girls, an interest in violent TV programs at age 8 leads to less aggression at age 19.

4. Bender (1959), in a study of children and adolescents who had killed, found that death wishes may be acted upon when:

a) Sibling rivalry becomes intensely severe due to some external factor, such as a child being placed outside the home because of the birth of a younger sibling.

b) Foster homes fail to give positive experiences of love and security to a child, or they repeat the rejection and deprivation he/she has suffered from biological parents.

c) Illness or congenital deficiencies make the child feel helpless and in need of greater love than he/she receives.

d) Educational difficulties, especially reading disabilities, make school adjustment difficult, and the child does not receive help or support from parents or teachers.

e) There is an identification by the child with aggressive adults and a family pattern of violent behavior.

5. Tooley (1975) reported on a boy and girl, both 6 years old,

who had tried to murder their younger siblings:

a) Both came from homes where the mothers tended to be childish and self-centered and frequently abandoned all the children without notice or explanation, leaving the violent child to care for younger siblings.

b) In one home, the father was unavailable. In the other, the father and mother were officially divorced but frequently got together. This father often physically abused the children while drinking.

c) Both children had a special relationship with their mother in which they saw themselves as her caretakers, thus helping the mother make her difficult life more tolerable for her.

d) The mothers were aware of and supported the relationship at the expense of the well-being of the younger siblings.

e) Each child was the only one in the family to act out with dangerous aggression.

f) The mothers unconsciously wished to be rid of all the children, and the aggressors were placed in the situation of assuring the mother's return by getting rid of the younger siblings.

EXAMINATION OF THE CHILD:

1. In Tooley's study, the aggressive 6-year-olds were noted to have the following characteristics:

a) They did not have a concept of death as irreversible, but did understand the meaning of present and absent, and had a barely suppressed wish to be rid of their younger siblings.

b) They lacked sadistic interest in inflicting pain.

c) They saw themselves in the role of special caretakers to the mothers and did not regard adults as protectors.

d) They were self-confident, convincing and attractive children.

e) They were constant, careful surveyors of their environment.

f) They had a generous supply of curiosity and made shrewd assessments of interpersonal situations.

g) Clinical examination led to the impression that they were very bright, but objective testing placed them in the average to high-average range.

h) Their aggressive acts involved firesetting, choking, and attempted drowning.

2. In older children and adolescents, there are fewer positive attributes:

a) While the child or adolescent may be superficially friendly, there is often an underlying intense anger and disregard for human values.

b) They distrust the environment, expecting to be harmed by any social interaction.

c) They may be hyperkinetic or have some physical abnormality.

d) They may consider the victim or potential victim as an obstructing object or a nonperson (King, 1975).

e) Their speech is loaded with action words and is likely to be provocative: "Fuck you!" "Make me!"

f) They are street-wise and appear intelligent but on formal testing show only average intelligence.

g) They often read below their grade level.

EXAMINATION OF THE PARENTS:

1. There may be physical evidence of violent behavior between the parents.

2. Alcoholism is common (King, 1975; Duncan and Duncan, 1971).

3. Children, in general, appear to be unwanted.

4. The parents frequently appear to get some pleasure from the child's aggressive behavior. This may be manifested by

a smile during the telling of an incident, or by minimizing its seriousness by saying, "I did that too, when I was a kid," or by intense interest in the child's aggressive behavior.

DIFFERENTIAL DIAGNOSIS:

1. Violent behavior can occur with any psychiatric disturbance. It is more common with sociopathic personalities, unsocialized aggressive reactions, group delinquent reactions, explosive personality disorders and paranoid schizophrenia. Violent attacks may occur with temporal lobe epilepsy, but Lewis (1975) has written that "no competent observer appears to have seen such an attack."

2. Several factors should be considered in the assessment of potential for violent behavior. Duncan lists the following seven criteria (Duncan and Duncan, 1971):

   a) "The intensity of the patient's hostile destructive impulses, as expressed verbally, behaviorally, or in psychometric test data. This assessment should include a detailed history of the patient's past life experiences.

   b) The patient's control over his impulses as determined by history and current behavior, particularly in response to stress

   c) The patient's knowledge of and ability to pursue realistic alternatives to a violent resolution of an untenable life situation. An apparently progressive development of explosive emotion accompanied by an attitude of hopelessness may warrant immediate intervention.

   d) The provocativeness of the intended victim and the patient's ability to cope with provocation currently and in the past

   e) The degree of helplessness of the intended victim

   f) The availability of weapons

   g) Homicidal hints or threats, which warrant serious concern if they are specific in regard to victim, means, details of fantasy, or measures to ensure escape"

3. Other factors (Hebert, 1977) which increase the risk of violence include:

   a) Anyone who has made homicidal preparations

   b) Paranoid patients who feel that the victim is trying to get them

   c) Schizophrenic patients hearing a voice telling them to kill someone

   d) Either person in a sadomasochistic relationship

   e) A schizophrenic mother with the child as a victim

   f) A person taking amphetamines or cocaine

4. Macdonald (1967) found that among those persons threatening homicide, the risk of homicide is higher in the absence of attempted suicide. Those who have attempted suicide are more likely to kill themselves than others.

IMMEDIATE TREATMENT:

1. Remind the patient of the difference between thought and deed. "It's OK to feel that way, but not OK to do it."

2. Attempt to separate the aggressor from the victim or provoking situation.

3. Appeal to the patient's narcissism and intelligence. "It's not very smart for a bright guy like you" or "If you can't pull the time, don't pull the crime."

4. Insist that the patient temporarily give up his/her weapons. If the patient has given up one weapon, it is wise to ask if he/she has another.

5. If sedation is indicated, avoid sedative hypnotics, including Valium, because a paradoxical effect or intoxication may occur.

6. Mellaril 50 mg/70 kg h. s. or up to t. i. d. may be used when oral medication is indicated. Haldol 5 mg/70 kg IM may be used when parenteral medication is needed (see Chapter V on psychopharmacology, p. 148).

7. When in doubt, admit the patient for observation, if necessary on an involuntary basis.

8. Attempt to warn the intended victim.

9. In the control of aggressive behavior, one should generally proceed from verbal control to physical control to chemical control.

10. If physical restraint becomes necessary, it is best to plan for its use ahead of time. If only two people are available, they should each take an arm and move the patient toward a secure room without trying to lift the patient. If the patient's weight is taken off his feet, he frequently begins kicking. If there are four people, one is assigned to each upper extremity, two are assigned to the lower extremities, and the patient is carried to a secure setting or placed in physical restraints.

11. Rosen and DiGiacomo (1978) offer several suggestions for the use of restraints:

    a) When the need for restraints is presented in a calm, yet firm, manner and the reasons and goals explained, many patients will cooperate willingly:

       (1) Restraints should be instituted in close temporal proximity to the behavior which necessitated their use.

       (2) If at all possible, the patient's primary caretaker should be present and take responsibility for this decision, or at least show concurrence.

    b) Physical force may be required when:

       (1) The staff has failed to respond to earlier signs of dyscontrol.

       (2) The need for restraints is presented in an ambivalent or hostile manner.

       (3) The decision to use and/or implement restraints occurs with staff who are not involved in the patient's care.

    c) If the patient must be placed in restraints involuntarily, the physician must immediately thereafter initiate the administrative process required for involuntary hospitalization.

    d) Leather or cloth bracelets are attached to the patient's limbs; then, by means of a belt, they are attached to the bed frame so the patient is maintained in a supine position.

e) Sufficient flexibility must be allowed so that the patient is able to move his/her limbs and roll on his/her side.

f) The bracelets must not be so tight that circulation is impaired. Foam rubber padding should be placed between cuffs and skin to prevent abrasions.

g) Once in restraints, the patient should be placed in a quiet, private room near the nursing station.

h) The decision to place the patient in restraints is an indication for increased, rather than decreased, observation and care:

   (1) Visits by the nursing staff should occur at least every fifteen minutes, and the patient should be helped in changing positions at hourly intervals.

   (2) If it is necessary for the patient to remain in restraints for over an hour or two, vital signs should be checked at least twice a day, and the patient should be assisted in eating and personal hygiene.

i) The patient is informed of improvement in his social, motor, affective and cognitive control and rewarded by increased privileges, such as the freeing of one arm or the use of cigarettes under supervision.

j) The primary focus of restraints is to foster the patient's sense of mastery by the graded return of responsibilities, such as bathroom privileges and meals.

12. The following scheme, which moves from internal to external control, may be used in teaching self-control of aggressive behavior:

a) Saying "stop it" to yourself (subvocally)
b) Saying "stop it" softly outloud
c) Saying "stop it" loudly
d) Having someone else say "stop it" softly
e) Having someone else say "stop it" loudly
f) Voluntarily isolating yourself (time out)
g) Voluntarily asking for medicine
h) Involuntary isolation (seclusion)
i) Involuntarily getting medicine
j) Voluntarily going into restraints
k) Involuntarily going into restraints

FOLLOW-UP TREATMENT:

1. Follow-up treatment depends upon the cause of the violent behavior and its severity:

   a) In one extreme, the youth's homicidal threat may have occurred after a great deal of stress, including a provocative victim. If the victim is no longer obtainable; the differences appear to be resolved; and there is no longer any homicidal ideation, then the patient might be rapidly discharged if the diagnosis is adjustment reaction.

   b) In the other extreme, if there is a long-standing history of serious violent behavior; an actual homicidal attempt with an unprovocative victim; and the diagnosis is psychosis, sociopathy, unsocialized aggressive reaction or impulse-ridden personality, then long-term treatment is often indicated. If the youth is not psychotic, he may be held responsible to legal charges before treatment can begin, or treatment may need to take place under the direction of the juvenile legal authority.

2. Long-term treatment should utilize a psychoeducational approach in which the child can work through, in psychotherapy, an intense anger at the world while relearning social and cognitive skills. Nearly all of these patients will need help in reading. There is some evidence that a training program in modeling and verbalization of cognitive activity to foster verbal mediation skills can be helpful. Teaching aggressive children to think aloud may help them with both cognitive and behavior problems (Camp, et al., 1977). Children and adolescents with hyperactivity may need adjunctive treatment with stimulant medication.

CHAPTER V

CHILD AND ADOLESCENT PSYCHOPHARMACOLOGY

GENERAL PRINCIPLES:

1. Prescribers' attitudes are important, since medication can often become part of the organic-dynamic-behaviorist polemic. A dynamic or behavioristically-oriented prescriber is likely to use homeopathic (very small) doses and, seeing no response, concludes that the medication is ineffective. The organically-oriented prescriber is likely to use medications inappropriately or at too great a dose and concludes that the medication is effective simply because the child is sedated.

2. Family attitudes can contribute to treatment results. If the family has heard about the medication from newspaper reports, or a friend or relative has taken it, their expectations will modify the drug's effect. Some families need to focus all difficulties on obscure organic causes and will often expect a miracle from medications. Thus, family expectations can either increase or decrease the effectiveness of any medication.

3. Patient attitudes affect drug response. Most children will readily accept medication if they feel it will help them and if the significant adults in their environment are supportive of their taking it. Adolescents often rebel, because medication threatens their emerging independence by confirming fears that they will be controlled by adults and will be seen as different by their peers. All patients have to understand that medication does not absolve them from taking responsibility nor solve all their behavior problems.

4. Realistic expectations include the following:

   a) Psychotropic medications do not entirely cure or eradicate the basic causes or consequences of any disorders.

   b) Improvement from medications can help the overall treatment by making parents realize that the problem can be helped.

c) Improvement can decrease parental guilt over feelings of total responsibility for the child's psychological problems.

d) In the severely disturbed, hyperactive, organic or functionally psychotic child, medication may mean the difference between outpatient management and institutionalization.

e) For most milder conditions, medications should be used as adjunctive treatment or not at all.

5. General techniques of administration include:

a) Select target behaviors for treatment.

b) Ask if any biological family member has used the same medication. A positive response by another family member adds to the indication for using that particular medication.

c) Start small and gradually increase the dose until a satisfactory response is obtained or side-effects limit the medication's usefulness. The maintenance dose should be the smallest effective dose, as side-effects may be dose-related.

d) Giving the medication on a once daily basis increases the probability that the patient will take the medication.

e) Drug holidays (no medications on weekends or vacations) give opportunities to observe whether use of the drug with the child is still necessary.

f) A white blood cell count should be obtained at the onset of treatment with major tranquilizers and periodically thereafter, because of the possibility of agranulocytosis.

6. "Drug therapy is almost always to be considered adjunctive and not the only or even the primary treatment. "(Wiener, 1977)

INDICATIONS FOR PSYCHOTROPIC MEDICATIONS:

Hyperkinetic Reaction or Attention Deficit Disorder (DSM III):

1. The diagnosis is based on the following cluster of symptoms:

a) Hyperactivity (not under volitional control and continues in inappropriate places, such as school and church)

b) Distractibility (any stimulus gets them going)

c) Impulsivity (unable to delay gratification)

d) Emotional lability (shows irritability and sudden fluctuations in mood with low frustration tolerance)

2. A modified form of Conners' check list (Conners, 1969) is widely available (Abbott Laboratories) and can be used, by the physician only, for screening (see Chapter VI, p. 156) as well as for following the child's progress:

a) The following items are scored on the parent's questionnaire:

(1) Excitable, impulsive
(2) Difficulty in learning
(3) Restless in the "squirmy" sense
(4) Restless, always "up and on the go"
(5) Denies mistakes or blames others
(6) Fails to finish things
(7) Childish or immature (wants help he shouldn't need; clings; needs constant reassurance)
(8) Distractibility or attention span a problem
(9) Mood changes quickly and drastically
(10) Easily frustrated in efforts

b) The following items are scored on the teacher's questionnaire:

(1) Restless in the "squirmy" sense
(2) Demands must be met immediately
(3) Distractibility or attention span a problem
(4) Disturbs other children
(5) Restless, always "up and on the go"
(6) Excitable, impulsive
(7) Fails to finish things that he starts
(8) Childish and immature
(9) Easily frustrated in efforts
(10) Difficulty in learning

c) The amount of behavior is scored according to four levels. Zero points are recorded for "not at all," one point for "just a little," two points for "pretty much," and three points for "very much." Scores above 15 on both questionnaires are an indication for further evaluation. After treatment has begun, the questionnaires can be given again to see if the score has been reduced.

3. Treatment with stimulant medications is only a part of the total treatment (see Chapter IV, p. 78 , for details on hyperkinesis):

a) Action: The onset is rapid (except with Cylert) and may be dramatic. A calmed, more integrated behavior pattern often results. There is improvement in cognitive functions, motor behavior, learning and school achievement. The attentional difficulties (with or without hyperactivity) are significantly reduced. It was formerly thought that most children outgrow the need for stimulant medications at puberty. Recent evidence indicates that this is untrue, that some hyperactive children will need to continue their medication through adolescence and a few even into adulthood (Mann and Greenspan, 1976).

b) Side-effects: Insomnia is usually seen early in treatment or when the medication is given after 4:00 P.M., but it may be due to a rebound from the medication wearing off or from too low a dose. Anorexia occurs but usually diminishes over the first month. Growth inhibition has been reported with both Dexedrine and Ritalin (Safer, et al., 1972) but was not seen on doses of 20 mg of Ritalin or less. Growth charts should be maintained on all children being given stimulant medications to monitor this side-effect. The amphetamine-look (pale face, dark circles under the eyes) is uncommon, does not represent serious toxicity and will disappear with a slight reduction in dose. Children receiving stimulant medications do not experience euphoria, and there is no evidence of increased risk of drug dependency in later life.

c) Specific medications:

(1) Dexedrine (dextroamphetamine sulphate) is the oldest medication in this class. Start with 5 mg in the morning or twice daily (morning and noon). Increase the total daily dose by 5 mg every week. Total doses which exceed 30 mg/day may have to be split. Dexedrine spansules can be used to avoid a b. i. d. dose because of their long action, but absorption may be erratic.

(2) Ritalin (methylphenidate hydrochloride) is the most commonly used medication in this class. Start with 10 mg, 30 minutes before breakfast, as food or milk in the stomach may inhibit absorption. Increase by 5-10 mg/day, every week. Since Ritalin is very short-acting, a morning and noon schedule is often

necessary at doses above 35 mg/day. Doses over 60 mg/day are not recommended. Ritalin is not approved by the FDA for children under age 6.

(3) Cylert (pemoline) is the newest medication in this class and is inherently long-acting. Start with 37.5 mg/day, in a single morning dose. Increase the dose by 18.5 mg/day, every week. Benefits may not be obvious for four weeks. Side-effects may appear before benefits.

4. Treatment with antidepressants (only if all of the previously mentioned medications are not effective): Tofranil (imipramine hydrochloride) is not FDA approved for children less than 12 years of age, except for the treatment of enuresis. It is generally thought to give a good initial response in children with hyperactivity, followed by a rapid decrease in effectiveness. There is a serious risk of death (most often due to cardiac arrhythmia) in overdose with Tofranil.

Behavior Disorders, Non-psychotic Anxiety or Agitation:

1. Medications are usually not indicated only for the first-line, long-term treatment of relatively benign disorders. They are commonly used in the behavior disorders, but the indications are clinical, not based on empirical research.

2. They are best used on a one-time crisis basis, or on a time-limited basis for the treatment of disabling situational anxiety.

3. The message to the child should be that the medication is to help gain some self-control, not as a punishment.

4. Treatment with sedating antihistamines:

a) Benadryl (diphenhydramine hydrochloride) can be used for children of all ages. Its sedation is similar to that of phenothiazines in that there is no euphoria. There is no addiction liability, and the medication may be given in high doses before significant side-effects are seen. It is available as 12.5 mg/5 ml elixir, 25 and 50 mg capsules and as an intramuscular preparation. The dose is 5 mg/kg/day, which may need to be exceeded before drowsiness appears. Benadryl is rapidly absorbed and has a short duration of action (four to six hours). At least one report (Fish, 1968) has shown good results for anxiety and irritability in children under the age of 10.

b) Atarax and Vistaril (hydroxyzine hydrochloride) are basically similar to Benadryl. They are available as 25 mg/5cc and 10 mg/5cc syrup and as 25, 50 and 100 mg capsules or tablets. The dose for children under 6 years of age is 50 mg/day, given in divided doses. For children over 6 years of age, 100 mg/day can be given in divided doses.

5. Treatment with sedative-hypnotics:

a) Valium (diazepam) is an unusually safe medication. There have been few reported deaths from overdoses of Valium alone. Reports of addiction in adults are increasing. It is rapidly and well absorbed orally with an onset of action in 30 minutes and a peak of action in four hours. It has a long duration of action that exceeds 24 hours. Begin with 2.5 mg b.i.d. and increase gradually. When the dose exceeds 10 mg/day, it can be given in a single daily dose. Intramuscular injections may be erratically absorbed; therefore, this medication should only be given PO or IV. There is no FDA approval for use in children under 6 years of age.

b) Barbiturates are contraindicated in children because of the paradoxical excitement in younger children and the high addiction liability in adolescents.

6. Treatment with major tranquilizers:

a) Early, uncontrolled reports gave uniformly positive results; however, more recent, controlled studies showed decreased learning and cognitive functioning.

b) Major tranquilizers can now be recommended only for the most severely disturbed children; autistic, schizophrenic and brain-damaged children; and adolescents (Conners, 1975).

Childhood Psychosis:

1. General comments on the use of major tranquilizers (Conners, 1975):

a) No firm relationship between diagnosis and clinical benefit has been shown except for adult-type schizophrenia. Major tranquilizers should be reserved for children with the most severe symptoms and used in conjunction with other treatment techniques.

b) Retarded schizophrenic children may tolerate larger doses than older, less impaired children. Target symptoms of poor motor skills, decreased social responsiveness and poor communicative language usually improve.

c) Assaultive and self-mutilating children, when treated with these medications, can often respond to educational and milieu treatment.

d) Start with the lowest recommended dose and gradually increase it over two to four weeks to establish efficacy. A common error is to maintain a child on small, ineffective or marginally effective doses.

e) The most common side-effect is lassitude, which usually decreases over a few days. The most disturbing side-effects are the dystonias (torticollis, dysphagia, oculogyric crisis), which occur early in treatment, rapidly respond to Benadryl, and seldom recur.

f) Although uncommon, tardive dyskinesias can appear on withdrawal. Dyskinesias appear in extremities as choreiform movements or as ataxia (as opposed to the buccal-oral symptoms of adults) and commonly disappear within 14 days after withdrawal, although some may persist for 3 to 12 months (McAndrew, et al., 1972).

g) Agranulocytosis is a rare side-effect. It does not appear to be dose-related. It usually appears in the first eight weeks of treatment and is heralded by sore throat and fever. If this occurs, a white cell count should immediately be obtained and the medication withheld. If the count is depressed, the medications are discontinued and a hematologic consultation obtained.

h) Controlled studies have not demonstrated any stimulating effects from the high potency major tranquilizers, despite the common clinical belief to the contrary.

2. Treatment with major tranquilizers:

a) Mellaril (thioridazine-low potency piperadine phenothiazine):

(1) The medication causes moderate to high sedation.

(2) Anticholinergic side-effects are common (dry mouth, lactation and genitourinary symptoms including delayed or retrograde ejaculation and impotence).

    (3) Extrapyramidal side-effects occur infrequently, and this is an important advantage of the use of this medication.

    (4) The dose for children age 5-12 is 30-300 mg/day. It is not available in an injectable form.

    (5) There is no FDA approval for children less than two years old. There is an absolute limit of 800 mg/day because of the possibility of retinitis pigmentosa.

b) Thorazine (chlorpromazine - low potency aliphatic phenothiazine):

    (1) This medication causes marked sedation.

    (2) Anticholinergic side-effects are moderate in frequency.

    (3) Extrapyramidal side-effects are moderate in frequency.

    (4) The dose for children from age 5-12 is 30-300 mg/day. For children over 12, the dose is 75-800 mg/day. Doses over 1000 mg/day may rarely be necessary.

    (5) It is not FDA approved for use in children under 6 months old.

c) Stelazine (trifluoperazine hydrochloride - high potency piperazine phenothiazine):

    (1) This medication causes moderate sedation.

    (2) Anticholinergic side-effects are moderate in frequency.

    (3) Extrapyramidal side-effects are frequent.

    (4) The dose for children under age 12 is 1-20 mg/day; for children over 12 the dose is 4-40 mg/day.

    (5) It is not FDA approved for use in children under 6 months old.

d) Prolixin (fluphenazine - high potency piperazine phenothiazine):

    (1)   The medication causes minimal sedation.

    (2)   Anticholinergic side-effects are moderate in frequency.

    (3)   There are frequent extrapyramidal side-effects.

    (4)   The dose for children under age 12 is 1-7. 5 mg/day; for children over 12, the dose is 2. 5-20 mg/day.

    (5)   It is FDA approved for use in children over the age of 6 (Campbell, 1977).

e) Haldol (haloperidol - high potency butyrophenone):

    (1)   The medication causes moderate sedation.

    (2)   An important advantage of this medication is that anticholinergic side-effects are infrequent.

    (3)   Extrapyramidal side-effects are very frequent in adults.

    (4)   The usual dose is from 0. 5 to 5 mg/day.

    (5)   It is not FDA approved for use with children under age 12.

    (6)   It is the most effective drug for the control of the tics and vocal utterances of Gilles de la Tourette's syndrome.

f) Navane (thiothixene - high potency thioxanthene):

    (1)   This medication causes the least sedation in adults. Data on children are incomplete. Navane is not recommended for children under age 12, nor is it FDA approved.

    (2)   Anticholinergic side-effects are low to moderate in frequency.

    (3)   Extrapyramidal side-effects are moderate to high in frequency.

    (4)   The dose for children over age 12 is 2 to 60 mg/day.

    (5)   Chronic adult schizophrenics showed an increased

work output when given this medication. There is no equivalent study in children.

3. Choice of medication is largely empirical. The physician should know one medication from each chemical class, and begin with the oldest and best known class, and give this medication an adequate trial (dose and time) before moving to another. If the child is not markedly agitated, the physician would begin with Prolixin or Stelazine then move to Navane and finally Haldol. If the child is markedly agitated the physician would begin with Thorazine or Mellaril then move to Taractan and finally Haldol. There is wide individual variation in dose requirements among children, but adolescents usually require adult doses.

Adolescent Schizophrenia:

1. General comments:

   a) In marked contrast to the use of medications in the treatment of childhood psychoses, large, cooperative, well-controlled studies have shown antipsychotic medications to be effective in the treatment of adult-type schizophrenia (May, 1968).

   b) May's study compared medication alone, medication and psychotherapy, psychotherapy alone and electroconvulsive therapy. All of the patients in this study also received milieu therapy.

   c) Medication alone, and psychotherapy plus medication were the most effective treatments. By clinical criteria the advantage was generally with psychotherapy plus medication. The largest advantage occurred in terms of the patients' insight into their illness. Statistically, these two groups were distinguishable only in terms of cost. Psychotherapy plus medication was very significantly more expensive.

   d) Psychotherapy alone and milieu therapy were clearly the least effective and the most expensive forms of treatment, with little to choose between them. ECT was not effective as either medication alone or medication plus psychotherapy. For developmental reasons, ECT should be a treatment of last resort in adolescents.

   e) There was no evidence of antagonism between medication and psychotherapy. By almost all the clinical and cost criteria, medication had a powerful, beneficial effect, while the effect of psychotherapy was nonsignificant.

2. Emergency treatment:

a) In the case of agitated patients, Haldol is the medication of choice, largely because patients can be calmed without undue side-effects, such as hypotension. If the patient is only moderately agitated and somewhat cooperative, and is unable to be calmed by psychosocial intervention alone, Haldol can be given as the concentrate, usually in an initial dose of 5 mg. It is tasteless and does not have the local anesthetic properties of the phenothiazines, a distinct advantage. Its tastelessness should not suggest an opportunity to give the medication surreptitiously, a method which is in especially poor taste in an adolescent setting. The medication is simply offered to the patient in a suitable container with orange juice or soda pop. The dose of 5 mg can be repeated in 30 minutes and can be raised to 10 mg if necessary. Thereafter, 5 to 10 mg can be given every hour as needed.

b) If the patient is moderately agitated but unwilling to take the medication in the form of a concentrate, and the milieu is unable to manage the patient without assistance from medications, antipsychotic medications, with the exception of Mellaril, can be given intramuscularly. Haldol again has an advantage. Its IM dose is the same as the oral dose, whereas the IM phenothiazine dose is 1/2 to 1/3 the oral dose. Hypotension is much more frequently reported for phenothiazines than for Haldol. As it is wise to remember the adolescent's self-esteem, the injection should take place away from the mainstream of the ward, preferably with the patient sitting in a chair while the injection is given in the deltoid muscle.

c) In the case of the patient who is severely agitated, combative or assaultive, a locked facility with adequate staffing is a minimum requirement. Adequate medication followed by a short period of time in a seclusion room (where the patient can be observed by the staff) is preferable to an angry ongoing staff-patient encounter, ending with the patient being restrained and perhaps having battered one or more staff members. These patients can be given an initial 5 mg dose of Haldol IM, followed by 10 mg in 30 minutes if there have been no untoward effects, and followed thereafter by 10 mg IM every hour until the patient is no longer assaultive. It is rare that a total of more than 30 mg needs to be given before the patient is considerably calmed. Recently, some clinicians have favored giving tremendous doses in the first hours of admission in order to effect an early discharge (in some cases the same day!). The long-term efficacy of this procedure awaits further proof, at best, and raises many questions.

d) The only disadvantage seen with Haldol is the very high incidence of extrapyramidal reactions. An unproven clinical aphorism is that these reactions seldom occur in the first hours of therapy; however, it seems wise to provide for the possibility. Haldol tends to produce dystonias and akathisias, both of which seem less responsive to the more usual antiparkinsonian agents like Cogentin than to Benadryl. Therefore, Benadryl 50-100 mg can be given orally or IM every 4 hours as necessary with a recommended daily limit of 300 mg. At times, up to 600 mg per day of Benadryl, or a reduction in the dose of Haldol, may be necessary to control these reactions.

3. Routine treatment or follow-up of emergency treatment:

a) Choice of medication (see Table V. 1):

(1) Except for Sparine (promazine hydrochloride) and Dartal (thiopropazate hydrochloride) which are inferior, the rest of the antipsychotics are equivalent in antipsychotic effectiveness (Klein and Davis, 1969). Therefore, the physician chooses the medication on the basis of common side-effects: sedation, extrapyramidal side-effects and hypotensive effects. Since there are many of these medications, it is best to know one medication from each chemical class well. Two recently introduced entities, Moban (molindone hydrochloride), and Loxitane (loxapine), have added little to the armamentarium, except that Moban has been shown to cause less weight gain in patients taking the medication over a period of time.

(2) The usual starting dose for a 70 kg individual is the equivalent of 200 mg of Thorazine daily. If daytime sedation is needed, the dose may be split. If the prescriber is concerned about idiosyncratic reactions, such as hypotension, a small amount, such as 25 mg Thorazine or its equivalent may be given; if no untoward effects are seen in two hours, the remainder may be given. The dose is increased by 100 to 200

TABLE V. 1: COMMON ANTIPSYCHOTIC DRUGS IN EQUIVALENT DOSES

SED	EPS	HT	DOSE (Mg)	MEDICATION	GROUP
H	M-P	M	100	Thorazine (chlorpromazine)	aliphatic phenothiazine
M	L-P	M	100	Mellaril (thioridazine)	piperadine phenothiazine
H	H-P	L	50	Vesprin (triflupromazine)	aliphatic phenothiazine
L	H-P, D	L	8	Trilafon (perphenazine)	piperadine phenothiazine
M	H-P, D	L	5	Stelazine (trifluoperazine)	piperadine phenothiazine
M	H-D	L	2	Prolixin (fluphenazine)*	piperadine phenothiazine
L	H-D	L	5-10	Navane (thiothixene)	thioxanthene
M	VH-D	L	2.5	Haldol (haloperidol)	butyrophenone
M	H-D	L	10	Moban (molindone)	dihydroindolone
M	H-P, D	M	10	Loxitane (loxapine)	dibenzoxazepine

*Prolixin Decanoate 25 mg IM every 10-14 days is a long-acting phenothiazine approximately equal to 5 mg oral Prolixin per day.

SED = Sedation; EPS = Extrapyramidal Symptoms; HT = Hypotension; VH = Very High; H = High; M = Moderate
L = Low; P = Parkinsonism or restlessness; D = Dystonias

mg daily to a level of about 600 mg Thorazine or its
mg equivalent. With more than moderate mood
swings, suspiciousness or psychotic thinking, the
dose may be increased to about 2000 mg equivalents.
Several VA studies have shown that increasing the
dose beyond about 1500 mg equivalents rarely makes
a difference in the patient's response (Prien and
Cole, 1968). Recently, some investigators have used
the high potency antipsychotics in very high doses,
for example, 5000 to 50,000 mg equivalents. This
method has not been studied sufficiently to be generally recommended.

(3)   The action of these medications is complex and includes reducing the motor arousal, reducing anxiety
and social withdrawal and clearing the thinking disorder of the patient. Lehmann (1966) has pointed out
that these symptoms tend to disappear in a certain
order. The symptoms of arousal, such as restlessness and insomnia, are resolved in two to four weeks.
Anxiety, hostility and social withdrawal decrease
after three to six weeks. The delusions and hallucinations of the thinking disorder may disappear only
after six to eight weeks, even though the patient may
no longer report them after a week.

(4)   The patient's symptoms come under control, according to the timetable as shown in item 3. It usually
takes four to eight weeks for complete remission. At
this point, the patient should be receiving all of his
daily dose at bedtime, unless a split dose is needed
for daytime sedation. Gradually, over a period of
weeks, the dose is reduced to about one-third to one-
half the amount used during the acute period or a
range of 75 to 300 mg Thorazine or its equivalent.
At this stage a common error is to discontinue medication too quickly, and a good practice is to have the
patient in remission for six months before reducing
the dose by one-third. If no deterioration is seen in
two months, another one-third of the dose can be decreased and again in another two months, so that in
about a year after an acute episode a patient can be
drug-free. Several studies have shown that as many
as three-fourths of schizophrenics will relapse within 12 months of being off all anti-psychotic medications, while only a third of those maintained on medication will relapse. However, the serious long-term
side-effects of tardive dyskinesia associated with the

use of these medications makes it imperative that all patients be given a trial without medication. Common side-effects of these medications are discussed earlier in this section on the treatment of childhood psychoses (see Chapter V, p. 144).

Depression:

1. The role of medication in the treatment of childhood depression is severely limited by the lack of consensus about diagnosis and by the lack of well-controlled studies. At this time in North America, the treatment of childhood depression seldom includes the use of medication. In Europe, antidepressant drugs are more commonly used (Frommer, 1967).

2. Depressions in adolescents which resemble adult endogenous depressions respond to tricyclic antidepressants. These depressions are characterized by gradual onset, weight loss, early morning or middle of the night sleep disturbance and a family history of serious depression.

3. Treatment by tricyclic antidepressants:

   a) Tofranil (imipramine hydrochloride):

   (1) This medication causes minimal or no sedation.

   (2) Anticholinergic effects are always seen with the use of therapeutic doses; the most common are dry mouth and blurred vision. Constipation and urinary retention are less frequently seen.

   (3) At very high doses (4 mg/kg and above), orthostatic hypotension and myoclonic jerks may appear, as well as EKG changes.

   (4) The minimal effective dose for adolescents is 2 mg/kg, beginning at small doses and increasing gradually. Much or all of the dose can be given at bedtime to minimize side-effects.

   (5) Single ingestions over 1000 mg are commonly fatal in adults, and recent reports indicate that 500 mg can cause serious life-threatening arrhythmias. Even smaller, single doses are dangerous in children, and therefore, only very small amounts should be prescribed. Routine inquiry should be made about suicidal ideation, and the drug should be prescribed only

on an inpatient basis if such thoughts are present.
In an overdose, the physician should aim to get the
drug out before it is absorbed. Once plasma-bound,
it is undialyzable. Conservative treatment is preferred in overdoses. Physostigmine should be used
only when serious side-effects, such as arrhythmias,
are present, and then only in the hands of a trained
clinician, since this drug can induce seizures (see
section on treatment of anticholinergic toxicity,
Chapter IV, p. 23).

Mania:

1. Treatment with lithium carbonate:

   a) Lithium has been known to be an effective antimanic agent
   since 1949. Several deaths resulted when it was used as
   a salt substitute in patients with congestive heart failure,
   and therefore, it did not come into general use until the
   1970's.

   b) The mechanism of action is unknown but is thought to involve inhibition of the sodium pump at the cellular level.

   c) Lithium carbonate is well absorbed orally, and a peak
   blood level occurs in one or two hours. About 95% of the
   lithium is excreted by the kidneys. If sodium intake is
   restricted, the amount of lithium resorbed is increased,
   so patients must be warned about dietary restriction of
   salt and use of diuretics which deplete sodium.

   d) Treatment is initiated only after adequate renal function
   is assessed by BUN and creatinine studies and baseline
   thyroid studies (T_3, T_4) are obtained. EKGs are obtained
   only if a physical exam shows some cardiac abnormality:

      (1) Begin with 900 mg/70 kg lithium carbonate the first
      day, in 3 divided doses, and increase to 1800 mg/70
      kg the next day.

      (2) Since the serum level rises rapidly in adolescents,
      doses of 2400 mg/70 kg a day seldom need to be ex-
      ceeded. Usually a level above 1.0 mEq/l can be
      achieved in 5 to 7 days.

      (3) Clinically, however, the adolescent does not respond
      any sooner than the adult, and the dose must be moni-
      tored carefully in the first five- to ten-day period to

avoid toxicity.

(4) Serum lithium levels are determined every Monday, Wednesday and Friday. Because rapid absorption quickly alters blood levels, the morning dose is held until the blood is drawn.

(5) Once the mania subsides, the dose is reduced by about one-half and the entire daily dose of up to 1200 mg may be given at bedtime.

e) Response to the lithium is judged by the patient's behavior, side-effects and serum lithium levels as indicated below:

(1) The patient's psychomotor agitation and disturbed mood gradually respond. Pacing and talking decrease, so that the patient no longer has to jump up to shake hands or make another request. Jocularity or irritability are replaced by solemnness. However, the patient may complain of being tired or depressed. The pressured speech slows so that he/she can carry on a normal conversation.

(2) Expect mild thirst and fine tremor as concomitants of therapy. Nausea or a feeling like seasickness are sometimes reported as the dose is increased or an hour or two after any dose. Protracted nausea, vomiting, diarrhea or lack of coordination are indications for withholding medication for 24 hours and then resuming treatment with a reduced dose.

(3) The serum lithium level reflects only indirectly the amount of lithium in the central nervous system. Levels between 1.0 and 1.5 mEq/l are usually necessary for the control of acute episodes. A range of 0.8 to 1.2 mEq/l is used for prophylactic treatment. Levels above 2.0 mEq/l are considered toxic, and the lithium should be stopped immediately. If the patient has serious signs of toxicity, such as a decreased consciousness or muscle fasciculations, supportive measures should be employed in consultation with an internist or pediatrician. Mannitol or aminophylline and an alkaline urine can be used to induce a lithium diuresis. (Fieve, 1975).

2. Treatment with major tranquilizers:

a) Major tranquilizers are used in moderate to severe mania or in milder mania if the patient refuses to take lithium carbonate, which is available only as an oral preparation.

b) They are useful only for the acute phase, since there is no evidence that they provide any prophylactic value in the low dose levels that would be used in the periods between acute episodes of mania.

c) They are frequently used in combination with lithium carbonate to provide control of manic behavior while the serum lithium concentration builds up.

d) Care must be taken to reduce the dose of major tranquilizers as lithium approaches therapeutic levels so that the patient is not unduly sedated.

e) Any major tranquilizer can be used:

   (1) Doses of 1000 mg/70 kg Thorazine, or its equivalent, may be necessary.

   (2) Haldol has been widely used, but there is no evidence that it is specifically useful in the treatment of acute mania.

3. Treatment with electroconvulsive therapy (ECT):

   a) ECT was the first treatment used for acute mania when sedative hypnotic medications were found to be ineffective.

   b) Currently, it should only be considered as the treatment of last resort for adolescents. Indications would require all three of the following criteria:

      (1) Patients who are severely manic and likely to do harm to themselves or others

      (2) Patients who are unwilling to take lithium carbonate

      (3) Patients who are unresponsive to or unable to use any major tranquilizers because of allergy or pregnancy

CHAPTER VI

PARENT AND TEACHER QUESTIONNAIRES

PARENT'S QUESTIONNAIRE

Name of Child _____ Date _____

Please answer all questions. Beside each item below, indicate the degree of the problem by a check mark (✓):

	Not at all	Just a little	Pretty much	Very much
1. Picks at things (nails, fingers, hair, clothing)				
2. Sassy to grown-ups				
3. Problems with making or keeping friends				
4. Excitable, impulsive				
5. Wants to run things				
6. Sucks or chews (thumb; clothing; blankets)				
7. Cries easily or often				
8. Carries a chip on his shoulder				
9. Daydreams				
10. Difficulty in learning				
11. Restless in the "squirmy" sense				

(Cont.)

	Not at all	Just a little	Pretty much	Very much
12. Fearful (of new situations; new people or places; going to school)				
13. Restless, always up and on the go				
14. Destructive				
15. Tells lies or stories that aren't true				
16. Shy				
17. Gets into more trouble than others of the same age				
18. Speaks differently from others of the same age (baby talk; stuttering; hard to understand)				
19. Denies mistakes or blames others				
20. Quarrelsome				
21. Pouts and sulks				
22. Steals				
23. Disobedient or obeys, but resentfully				
24. Worries more than others (about being alone; illness or death)				
25. Fails to finish things				
26. Feelings easily hurt				
27. Bullies others				

(Cont.)

	Not at all	Just a little	Pretty much	Very much
28. Unable to stop a repetitive activity				
29. Cruel				
30. Childish or immature (wants help he shouldn't need; clings; needs constant reassurance)				
31. Distractibility or attention span a problem				
32. Headaches				
33. Mood changes quickly and drastically				
34. Doesn't like or doesn't follow rules or restrictions				
35. Fights constantly				
36. Doesn't get along well with brothers or sisters				
37. Easily frustrated in efforts				
38. Disturbs other children				
39. Basically an unhappy child				
40. Problems with eating (poor appetite; gets up between bites)				
41. Stomachaches				

(Cont.)

	Not at all	Just a little	Pretty much	Very much
42. Problems with sleep (can't fall asleep; up too early; up in the night)				
43. Other aches and pains				
44. Vomiting or nausea				
45. Feels cheated in family circle				
46. Boasts and brags				
47. Lets self be pushed around				
48. Bowel problems (frequently loose; irregular habits; constipation)				

The Hyperkinesis Index is based on a questionnaire developed by C. Keith Conners, Ph. D.

Distributed by Abbott Laboratories, North Chicago, IL 60064

TEACHER'S QUESTIONNAIRE

Name of Child _____ Date _____

Please answer all questions. Beside each item, indicate the degree of the problem by a check mark (✓):

	Not at all	Just a little	Pretty much	Very much
1. Restless in the "squirmy" sense				
2. Makes inappropriate noises when he shouldn't				
3. Demands must be met immediately				
4. Acts "smart" (impudent or sassy)				
5. Temper outbursts and unpredictable behavior				
6. Overly sensitive to criticism				
7. Distractibility or attention span a problem				
8. Disturbs other children				
9. Daydreams				
10. Pouts and sulks				
11. Mood changes quickly and drastically				

(Cont.)

	Not at all	Just a little	Pretty much	Very much
12. Quarrelsome				
13. Submissive attitude toward authority				
14. Restless, always up and on the go				
15. Excitable, impulsive				
16. Excessive demands for teacher's attention				
17. Appears to be unaccepted by group				
18. Appears to be easily led by other children				
19. No sense of fair play				
20. Appears to lack leadership				
21. Fails to finish things that he starts				
22. Childish and immature				
23. Denies mistakes or blames others				
24. Does not get along well with other children				
25. Uncooperative with classmates				
26. Easily frustrated in efforts				
27. Uncooperative with teacher				

(Cont.)

	Not at all	Just a little	Pretty much	Very much
28. Difficulty in learning				

The Hyperkinesis Index is based on a questionnaire developed by C. Keith Conners, Ph. D.

Distributed by Abbott Laboratories, North Chicago, IL 60064

CUESTIONARIO PARA LOS PADRES

Nombre del Nino _____ Fecha_____

Sirvase contestar todas las preguntas. Al lado de cade pregunta, indique con un signo (√) la gravedad del problema:

	No, en absoluto	Un poco	Bas-tante	Muchi-simo
1. Pizca (las unas, los dedos, los pelos, la ropa)				
2. Es insolente con las personas mayores				
3. Le resulta dificil hacer amigos o man-tenerlos				
4. Es excitable, impul-sivo				
5. Quiere dirigirlo todo				
6. Chupa o muerde (el pulgar; la ropa; las cobijas)				
7. Llora facil o fre-cuentemente				
8. Se deja provocar facilmente				
9. Sueña despierto				
10. Le resulta dificil aprender				

(Cont.)

	No en absoluto	Un poco	Bas- tante	Muchi- simo
11. Se retuerce y es inquieto				
12. Es miedoso (teme nuevas situaciones, nuevas personas o lugares, la escuela)				
13. Es intranquilo, siempre se levanta y se mueve				
14. Es destructivo				
15. Miente o cuenta cosas que no son ciertas				
16. Es timido				
17. Su conducta le causa mas problemas que la de otros ninos de la misma edad				
18. Habla distinto de otros ninos de igual edad (habla como bebe chiquito; tartamudea; dificil de entender)				
19. Niega equivocarse y acusa a los demas				
20. Es peleador				
21. Suele estar malhumorado y enfadado				
22. Hurta				
23. Desobedece u obedece de mala gana				

(Cont.)

	No en absoluto	Un poco	Bas- tante	Muchi- simo
24. Se inquieta mas que otros (al estar solo; ante la enfermedad o la muerta)				
25. No acaba nunca las cosas				
26. Se ofende facilmente				
27. Intimida a los demas				
28. Le cuesta interrumpir una accion repetitiva				
29. Es cruel				
30. Es aninado o inma- duro (pide ayuda que no deberia necesitar; se prende a la falda de la mama; siempre necesita que lo tran- quilicen)				
31. Es distraido o incapaz de concentrarse				
32. Tiene dolores de ca- beza				
33. Presenta frecuentes o bruscos cambios de humor				
34. No le gusta la disci- plina ni las restric- ciones, y no lo acepta				
35. Pelea constantemente				
36. No se entiende con sus hermanos o hermanas				

(Cont.)

	No en absoluto	Un poco	Bas-tante	Muchi-simo
37. A menudo queda desalentado en sus esfuerzos				
38. Molesta a los otros ninos				
39. Es basicamente desdichado				
40. Tiene problemas al comer (falta de apetito; se levanta despues de cada bocado)				
41. Tiene dolores de estomago				
42. Tiene dificultades para dormir (no logra dormirse; se levanta demasiado temprano; se levanta de noche)				
43. Tiene otros dolores y malestares				
44. Tiene vomitos o nausea				
45. No se siente parte de la familia				
46. Le gusta hacer alarde de si mismo				
47. Deja que otros le maltraten				
48. Tiene problemas de evacuacion (diarrea; se va al bano irregularmente; es constipado				

(Cont.)

El Indice de Hiperkinesis esta basado sobre un cuestionario for-mulado por C. Keith Conners, Ph. D.

Distribuido por Abbott Laboratories, North Chicago, IL 60064

BIBLIOGRAPHY

GENERAL PRINCIPLES OF
EMERGENCY ROOM EVALUATION

Despert, L. J.: Technical approaches used in the study and treatment of emotional problems in children. Psychiat Quart 11: 677-696, 1937.

Gross, H. and Herbert, M.: The effect of race and sex on variation of diagnosis and disposition in a psychiatric emergency room. J Nerv Ment Dis 148: 638-642, 1969.

Jackson, A. M., et al.: Race as a variable affecting the treatment of children. J Am Acad Child Psychia 13: 20-31, 1974.

Prugh, D. G.: Procedure Manual for the Children's Psychiatric Clinic, Division of Child Psychiatry, Department of Psychiatry, University of Colorado Medical Center. Unpublished manuscript, University of Colorado Medical Center, 1963.

Warren, R. C., et al.: Differential attitudes of black and white patients toward treatment in a child guidance clinic. Am J Orthopsychia 43: 384-393, 1973.

PSYCHIATRIC EMERGENCIES IN CHILDHOOD

Burks, H. L. and Hoekstra, M.: Psychiatric emergencies in children. AM J Orthopsychia 34: 134-137, 1964.

Mattsson, A., et al.: Suicidal behavior as a child psychiatric emergency. Archives Gen Psychia 20: 100-109, 1969.

Morrison, G. C.: Therapeutic intervention in a child psychiatry emergency service. J Am Acad Child Psychia 8: 542-558, 1969.

Morrison, G. C. and Collier, J. G.: Family treatment approaches to suicidal children and adolescents. J Am Acad Child Psychia 8: 140-153, 1969.

SPECIFIC CHILD PSYCHIATRIC EMERGENCIES

ACUTE DRUG ABUSE:

Beebe, J. E. , III. : Evaluation and Treatment of the Drinking Patient. In: C. P. Rosenbaum and J. E. Beebe, III. (Eds.). Psychiatric Treatment: Crisis, Clinic, Consultation. New York: McGraw Hill, 1975, pp. 115-144.

Brecher, E. M. : Licit and Illicit Drugs. Boston: Little, Brown and Co. , 1972.

Cohen, S. : Glue sniffing. JAMA 231: 653-654, 1975.

Cohen, S. (Ed.): Alcohol - drug combinations. Drug Abuse & Alcohol Newsl 6: 1, Oct. , 1977.

Dilts, S. A. Hydroxyzine in the treatment of alcohol withdrawal. Am J Psychia 134: 92-93, 1977.

DuPont, R. L. Letter to State Mental Health Authorities on Phencyclidine Abuse. Department of Health, Education and Welfare, Rockville, Md. , Dec. 6, 1977.

Goldbert, T. M. , et al. : Comparative evaluation of treatments of alcohol withdrawal syndromes. JAMA 201: 113-116, 1967.

Granacher, R. P. and Baldessarini, R. J. : Physostigmine; its use in acute anticholinergic syndrome with antidepressant and antiparkinson drugs. Arch Gen Psychia 32: 375-380, 1975.

Jones, K. L. and Smith, D. W. : Recognition of the fetal alcohol syndrome in early infancy. Lancet 2: 999-1001, 1973.

Kaim, S. , et al. : Treatment of the acute alcohol withdrawal state: a comparison of four drugs. Am J Psychia 125: 1640-1646, 1969.

Showalter, C. V. and Thornton, W. E. : Clinical pharmacology of phencyclidine toxicity. Am J Psychia 134: 1234-1238, 1977.

Smith, D. E. and Wesson, D. R. : Phenobarbital technique for treatment of barbiturate dependence. Arch Gen Psychia 24: 56-60, 1971.

Thomas, D. W. and Freedman, D. X.: Treatment of the alcohol withdrawal syndrome. JAMA 188: 316-318, 1964.

Victor, M.: Treatment of the neurological complications of alcoholism. Modern Treatment 3: 491-501, 1968.

ADOLESCENT SCHIZOPHRENIA:

Babgigian, H. M.: Schizophrenia: Epidemiology. In: A. M. Freedman, H. I. Kaplan and B. J. Sadock (Eds.). Comprehensive Textbook of Psychiatry, 2nd Edition. Baltimore: Williams and Wilkins Co. , 1975, pp. 860-866.

Bateson, G. , et al. Toward a theory of schizophrenia. Behav Sci 1:251-264, 1956.

Davis, J. M. Overview: maintenance therapy in psychiatry: I. schizophrenia. Am J Psychia 132: 1237-1245, 1975.

Davis, J. M.: Recent developments in the drug treatment of schizophrenia. Am J Psychia 133: 208-213, 1976.

Feighner, J. P. , et al.: Diagnostic criteria for use in psychiatric research. Arch Gen Psychia 26: 57-63, 1972.

Lehmann, H. E.: Schizophrenia: Clinical Features. In: A. M. Freedman, H. I. Kaplan and B. J. Sadock (Eds.). Comprehensive Textbook of Psychiatry, 2nd Edition. Baltimore: Williams and Wilkins Co. , 1975, pp. 851-860.

May, P. R.: Schizophrenia: Evaluation of Treatment Methods. In: A. M. Freedman, H. I. Kaplan and B. J. Sadock (Eds.). Comprehensive Textbook of Psychiatry, 2nd Edition, Baltimore: Williams and Wilkins Co. , 1975, pp. 955-982.

May, P. R.: Rational treatment for an irrational disorder. Am J Psychia 133: 1008-1112, 1976.

Pincus, J. H. and Tucker, G. J.: Behavioral Neurology. New York: Oxford University Press, 1978.

Singer, M. T. and Wynne, L. C.: Differentiating characteristics of parents of childhood schizophrenics, childhood neurotics and young adult schizophrenics. Am J Psychia 120: 234-243, 1963.

Slater, E. , et al. : The schizophrenia-like psychoses of epilepsy. Brit J Psychia 109: 95-150, 1963.

Van Putten, T. Milieu therapy: contraindications? Arch Gen Psychia 29: 640-643, 1973.

Weiner, H. : Schizophrenia: Etiology. In: A. M. Freedman, H. I. Kaplan and B. J. Sadock (Eds.). Comprehensive Textbook of Psychiatry, 2nd Edition. Baltimore: Williams and Wilkins Co. , 1975, pp. 866-890.

Zubin, J. et al. : An Experimental Approach to Projective Techniques. New York: John Wiley and Sons, Inc. , 1965.

ANOREXIA NERVOSA:

Blinder, B. J. , et al. : Behavior therapy of anorexia nervosa. Am J Psychia 126: 1093-1098, 1970.

Bliss, E. : Anorexia Nervosa. In: A. M. Freedman, H. I. Kaplan and B. J. Sadock (Eds.). Comprehensive Textbook of Psychiatry, 2nd Edition. Baltimore: Williams and Wilkins Co. , 1975, pp. 1655-1660.

Bruch, H. Psychotherapy in primary anorexia nervosa. J Nerv Ment Dis 150: 51-67, 1970.

Bruch, H. : Eating Disorders: Obesity, Anorexia Nervosa, and the Person Within. New York: Basic Books, 1973.

Galdston, R. : Mind over matter: observations on 50 patients hospitalized with anorexia nervosa. J Am Acad Child Psychia 13: 246-263, 1974.

Liebman, R. , et al. : The role of the family in the treatment of anorexia nervosa. J Am Acad Child Psychia 13: 264-273, 1974.

CHILD ABUSE:

Blager, F. and Martin, H. : Speech and Language of Abused Children. In: H. Martin (Ed.). The Abused Child: A Multidisciplinary Approach to Developmental Issues and Treatment. Cambridge: Ballinger Publishing Co. , 1976, pp. 83-92.

Coppolillo, H. P.: Drug impediments to mothering behavior. Inter J Addict Dis 2: 201-208, 1975.

Helfer, R. E.: The Responsibility and Role of the Physician. In: R. E. Helfer and C. H. Kempe (Eds.). The Battered Child, 2nd Edition, Chicago: University of Chicago Press, 1974, pp. 25-39.

Holter, J. C. and Friedman, S. B. Child abuse: early case finding in the emergency department. Pediatrics 42: 128-138, 1968.

Kempe, C. H., et al.: The battered child syndrome. JAMA 181: 17-24, 1962.

Schmitt, B. D. and Kempe, C. H.: The pediatricians' role in child abuse. Curr Probl Pediat 5: 3-47, 1975.

Steele, B. F. and Pollock, C. B.: A Psychiatric Study of Parents who Abuse Infants and Small Children. In: R. E. Helfer and C. H. Kempe (Eds.). The Battered Child, 2nd Edition. Chicago: University of Chicago Press, 1974, pp. 89-133.

Thomas, A., et al.: Temperament and Behavior Disorders in Children. New York: New York University Press, 1968.

Thomas, A. and Chess, S.: Temperament and Development. New York: Brunner/Mazel, Inc., 1977.

CHILDHOOD PSYCHOSES:

Beres, D.: Ego deviation and the concept of schizophrenia. Psychoanal Study Child 11: 164- 235, 1956.

Miller, R. T.: Childhood schizophrenia: a review of selected literature. Inter J Ment Health 3: 3-46, 1973.

Rank, B.: Intensive Study and Treatment of Preschool Children who Show Marked Personality Deviations or "Atypical Development," and their Parents. In: G. Caplan (Ed.). Emotional Problems of Early Childhood. New York: Basic Books, pp. 491-501, 1955.

Rutter, M.: Concepts of autism: a review of research. J Child Psychol Psychia 9: 1-25, 1968.

Childhood Schizophrenia:

Creak, M.: Schizophrenic syndrome in childhood: further progress report (April 1964) of a working party. Dev Med Child Neurol 6: 530-535, 1964.

DeMyer, M., et al. Comparison of five diagnostic systems for childhood schizophrenia and infantile autism. J Autism Child Schizo 1: 175-189, 1971.

Hingtgen, J. N. and Bryson, C. Q.: Recent developments in the study of early childhood psychoses: infantile autism, childhood schizophrenia, and related disorders. Schizo Bul 5: 8-54, 1972.

Kolvin, I., et al.: Studies in the childhood psychoses, II. Brit J Psychia 118: 385-395, 1971.

Rutter, M.: Childhood schizophrenia reconsidered. J Autism Child Schizo 2: 315-337, 1972.

Early Infantile Autism:

Bettelheim, B.: The Empty Fortress: Infantile Autism and the Birth of the Self. New York: Free Press, 1967.

Birch, H. and Hertzig, M.: Etiology of schizophrenia: an overview. In: Proceedings of the first Rochester international conference. Excerpta Medica International Congress Series No. 151: 92-110, 1967.

DeMyer, M., et al.: Prognosis in autism: a follow-up study. J Autism Child Schizo 3: 199-246, 1973.

Eisenberg, L.: The autistic child in adolescence. Am J Psychia 112: 607-612, 1956.

Eisenberg, L.: The course of childhood schizophrenia. Arch Neurol Psychia 78: 69-83, 1957.

Fish, B., et al.: The Prediction of Schizophrenia in Infancy. In: P. H. Hock and J. Zubin (Eds.). Psychopathology of Schizophrenia. New York: Grune and Stratton, 1966, pp. 335-365.

Frank, G.: The role of the family in the development of psychopathology. Psycholog Bul 64: 191-205, 1965.

Kanner, L.: Autistic disturbances of affective contact. Nervous Child 2: 217-250, 1943.

Mahler, M. and Furer, M.: Child psychosis: a theoretical statement and its implications. J Autism Child Schizo 2: 213-218, 1972.

O'Gorman, C.: The Nature of Childhood Autism. London: Butterworths, 1970.

Ornitz, E. M. and Ritvo, E. R. Perceptual inconstancy in early infantile autism. Archives Gen Psychia 18: 76-98, 1968.

Reichler, R. and Schopler, E.: Observations on the nature of human relatedness. J Autism Child Schizo 1: 283-295, 1971.

Reiser, D.: Psychosis in infancy and early childhood, as manifested by children with atypical development. New Eng J Med 269: 790-798, 844-850, 1963.

Rimland, B.: Infantile Autism. New York: Appleton-Century-Crofts, 1964.

Rutter, M. , et al.: A five- to fifteen-year follow-up study of infantile psychosis. 2. Social and behavioral outcome. Brit J Psychia 113: 1183-1199, 1967.

Schopler, E. and Reichler, R.: Parents as cotherapists in the treatment of psychotic children. J Autism Child Schizo 1: 87-102, 1971.

Szurek, S. and Berlin, I. (Eds.). Clinical Studies in Childhood Psychoses. New York: Brunner/Mazel, Inc. , 1973.

Tustin, F.: Autism and Childhood Psychosis. London: Hogarth Press, 1972.

Wing, L. and Wing, J.: Multiple impairments in early childhood autism. J Autism Child Schizo 1: 256-266, 1971.

Symbiotic Psychosis or Interactional Psychosis:

Bergman, A.: "I and You": The Separation-Individuation Process in the Treatment of a Symbiotic-Psychotic Child. In: J. B. McDevitt and C. F. Settlage (Eds.). Separation-Individuation: Essays in Honor of Margaret S. Mahler. New York: International Universities Press, pp. 325-355, 1971.

Furer, M.: The development of a preschool symbiotic boy. Psychoanal Study Child 19: 448-469, 1964.

Mahler, M.: On child psychosis and schizophrenia: Autistic and symbiotic-infantile psychoses. Psychoanal Study Child 7: 286-305, 1952.

Mahler, M. S. and Furer, M.: Observations on research regarding the 'symbiotic syndrome' of infantile psychosis. Psychoanal Q 29: 317-327, 1960.

Mahler, M. S., et al.: The Psychological Birth of the Human Infant: Symbiosis and Individuation. New York: Basic Books, 1975.

Schizophreniform Psychosis:

Group for the Advancement of Psychiatry, Committee on Child Psychiatry. Psychopathological disorders in childhood: theoretical considerations and a proposed classification. New York: Group for the Advancement of Psychiatry, (GAP report, no. 62), 1966.

Jordan, K. and Prugh, D. G.: Schizophreniform psychosis of childhood. Am J Psychia 128: 323-331, 1971.

Manic-Depressive Illness:

Anath, J. and Pecknold, J. C.: Prediction of lithium response in affective disorders. J Clin Psychia 39: 95-100, 1978.

Anthony, E. J. and Scott, P.: Manic-depressive psychoses in childhood. J Child Psychol Psychia 1: 53-72, 1960.

Arieti, S.: Affective Disorders: Manic-Depressive Psychosis and Psychotic Depression. In: S. Arieti (Ed.). American Handbook of Psychiatry, (2nd Edition), Vol. 3, Adult Clinical Psychiatry. New York: Basic Books, pp. 449-490, 1974.

Carlson, G. A., et al.: A comparison of outcome in adolescent and late-onset bipolar manic-depressive illness. Am J Psychia 134: 919-922, 1977.

Carlson, G. A. and Strober, M.: Manic-depressive illness in early adolescence: a study of clinical and diagnostic characteristics in six cases. J Am Acad Child Psychia 17: 138-153, 1978.

Cohen, M. B., et al.: An intensive study of twelve cases of manic-depressive psychosis. Psychiatry 17: 103-122, 1954.

Cohen, R. A.: Manic-Depressive Illness. In: A. M. Freedman, H. I. Kaplan, & B. J. Sadock (Eds.). Comprehensive Textbook of Psychiatry, 2nd Edition. Baltimore: Williams and Wilkins Co., pp. 1012-1024, 1975.

Feighner, J. P., et al.: Diagnostic criteria for use in psychiatric research. Arch Gen Psychia 26: 57-63, 1972.

Feinstein, S. C. and Wolpert, E. A.: Juvenile manic-depressive illness. J Am Acad Child Psychia 12: 123-136, 1973.

Gilbert, J.: Clinical Psychological Tests in Psychiatric and Medical Practice. Springfield: Charles C Thomas, 1969.

Hebert, F. B.: Manic-Depressive Illness Underlying Marijuana Intoxication. Unpublished manuscript, 1978.

Horowitz, H. A. Lithium and the treatment of adolescent manic-depressive illness. J Nerv Ment Dis 38: 480-483, 1977.

Kessler, S.: Psychiatric Genetics. In: S. Arieti (Ed.). American Handbook of Psychiatry, 2nd Edition, Vol. 6, New Psychiatric Frontiers. New York: Basic Books, pp. 352-384, 1975.

Kraeplin, E.: Manic-Depressive Insanity and Paranoia. Edinburgh: E. S. Livingston, 1921.

McKnew, D. H. Jr., et al.: Clinical and biochemical correlates of hypomania in a child. J Am Acad Child Psychia 13: 576-585, 1974.

Winokur, G., et al.: Depressive disease, a genetic study. Arch Gen Psychia 24: 135-144, 1971.

Hysterical Psychosis:

Hollender, M. H. and Hirsch, S. J.: Hysterical psychosis. Am J Psychia 120: 1066-1074, 1964.

Siomopoulis, V.: Hysterical psychosis: psychopathological aspects. Brit J Med Psychol 44: 95-100, 1971.

Folie A Deux:

Coleman, S. and Last, S. A study of folie a deux. Journal of Mental Science 85:1212-1223, 1939.

Lasegue, C. and Falret, J.: (1877): La folie a deux. Translated by R. Michaud. Am J Psychia 121: 1-23, 1964.

DELIRIUM:

Adams, R. D. and Victor, M.: Derangements of Intellect and Behavior Including Delirium and Other Confusional States, Korsakoff's Amnestic Syndrome and Dementia. In: T. R. Harrison, et al. (Eds.). Principles of Internal Medicine. New York: McGraw-Hill, 1966, pp. 264-280.

Engel, G. L. and Romano, J.: Delirium, a syndrome of cerebral insufficiency. J Chron Dis 9: 260-277, 1959.

DEPRESSION:

Glaser, K.: Masked depression in children and adolescents. Am J Psychother 21: 565-574, 1967.

Poznanski, E. and Zrull, J. P.: Childhood depression: Clinical characteristics of overtly depressed children. Arch Gen Psychia 23: 8-15, 1970.

Rie, H. E.: Depression in childhood: a survey of some pertinent contributions. J Amer Acad Child Psychia 5: 653-685, 1966.

Spitz, R. A. and Wolf, K. M.: Anaclitic depression: an inquiry into genesis of psychiatric conditions in early childhood, II: Psychoanal Study Child 2: 313-342, 1946.

Toolan, J. M. Suicide and suicidal attempts in children and adolescents. Am J Psychia 118: 719-724, 1962.

THE DYING CHILD:

Binger, C. M. et al.: Childhood leukemia: emotional impact on patient and family. New Eng J Med 280: 414-418, 1969.

Gardner, G.: Childhood, death and human dignity: hypnotherapy for David. Internat J Clin Exper Hypnosis 24: 122-139, 1976.

Grollman, E. A. (Ed.): Explaining Death to Children. Boston: Beacon Press, 1967.

Nagera, H.: Children's reaction to the death of important objects: a developmental approach. Psychoanal Study Child 25:

360-400, 1970.

Nagy, M.: The child's theories concerning death. J Genetic Psychol 73: 3-27, 1948.

Richmond, J. B. and Waesman, H. A.: Psychologic aspects of management of children with malignant diseases. Am J Dis Children 89: 42-47, 1955.

Solnit, A. J. and Green, M.: The Pediatric Management of the Dying Child: Part II. The Child's Reaction to the Fear of Dying. In: A. J. Solnit and S. A. Provence (Eds.). Modern Perspectives in Child Development. New York: International Universities Press, 1963, pp. 217-228.

GILLES DE LA TOURETTE'S DISEASE (Maladie Des Tics):

Bruun, R. D. and Shapiro, A. K.: Differential diagnosis of Gilles de la Tourette's syndrome. J Nerv Ment Dis 155: 328-334, 1972.

Brunn, R. D., et al.: A follow-up of 78 patients with Gilles de la Tourette's syndrome. Arch Gen Psychia 133: 944-947, 1976.

Golden, G. S.: Tourette syndrome - the pediatric perspective. Am J Dis Children 131: 531-534, 1977.

Kelman, D. H. Gilles de la Tourette's disease in children: a reivew of the literature. J Child Psychol Psychia 6: 219-226, 1965.

Shapiro, A. K., et al.: Treatment of Tourette's syndrome with haloperidol, review of 34 cases. Arch Gen Psychia 28: 92-97, 1973.

Woodrow, K. M.: Gilles de la Tourette's disease: a review. Am J Psychia 131: 1000-1003, 1974.

GROUP HYSTERIA:

Caulfield, E.: Pediatric aspects of the Salem witchcraft tragedy: a lesson in mental health. Am J Dis Children 65: 788-802, 1943.

Schuler, E. A. and Parenton, V. J.: A recent epidemic of hysteria in a Louisiana high school. J Soc Psychol 17: 221-235, 1943.

HYPERKINETIC SYNDROME:

Farley, G. K. and Blom, G. E.: Mental Health Consultation to Schools. In: L. Mann and D. A. Sabatino (Eds.). Third Review of Special Education. New York: Grune and Stratton, 1976, pp. 1-18.

Fish, B.: The "one child, one drug" myth of stimulants in hyperkinesis: importance of diagnostic categories in evaluating treatment. Arch Gen Psychia 25: 193-203, 1971.

Schmitt, B. D., et al.: The hyperactive child. Clin Pediat 12: 154-169, 1973.

Werry, J.: Developmental hyperactivity. Pediat Clin N Amer 15: 581-599, 1968.

HYSTERIA:

Freud, S. (1896): The Aetiology of Hysteria. Standard Edition, Vol. 3. London: Hogarth Press, 1962.

Proctor, J. T.: Hysteria in childhood. Am J Orthopsychia 23: 394-407, 1958.

Proctor, J. T.: The Treatment of Hysteria in Childhood. In: M. Hammer and A. M. Kaplan (Eds.). The Practice of Psychotherapy with Children. Homewood, Ill.: Dorsey Press, 1967.

Veith, I.: Hysteria: The History of a Disease. Chicago: University of Chicago Press, 1965.

REACTIONS TO ILLNESS, HOSPITALIZATION AND SURGERY:

Adams, M. S.: A hospital play program: helping children with serious illness. Am J Orthopsychia 46: 416-424, 1976.

Bergmann, T. and Freud, A.: Children in the Hospital. New York: International Universities Press, 1966.

Cassell, S. and Paul, M.: The role of puppet therapy on the emotional response of children hospitalized for cardiac catheterization. J Pediat 71: 233-239, 1967.

Mason, E. A.: The hospitalized child - his emotional needs. New Eng J Med 292: 406-414, 1965.

Petrillo, M. and Sanger, S.: Emotional Care of Hospitalized Children. Philadelphia: J. B. Lippincott Co., 1970.

Plank, E. N.: Working with Children in Hospitals, 2nd Edition. Cleveland: Press of Case Western Reserve, 1972.

Prugh, D. G. and Eckhardt, L. O.: Children's Reaction to Illness, Hospitalization and Surgery. In: A. M. Freedman, H. I. Kaplan and B. J. Sadock (Eds.). Comprehensive Textbook of Psychiatry, 2nd Edition. Baltimore: Williams and Wilkins Co., 1975, pp. 2100-2107.

Robertson, J.: Young Children in Hospitals, 2nd Edition. London: Tavistock Publications, Ltd., 1970.

Schowalter, J. E. and Lord, R. D.: Utilization of patient meetings on an adolescent ward. Psychia Med 1: 197-206, 1970.

Wolinsky, F. G.: Materials to prepare children for hospital experience. Except Child 37: 527-528, 1971.

RUNAWAY CHILDREN:

Jenkins, R. L.: The runaway reaction. Am J Psychia 128: 163-173, 1971.

Meeks, J.: The Fragile Alliance: An Orientation to the Outpatient Psychotherapy of the Adolescent. Baltimore: Williams and Wilkins Co., 1971.

Raphael, M. and Wolf, J.: Runaways. New York: Drake Publishers, 1974.

Stierlin, H.: A family perspective on adolescent runaways. Arch Gen Psychia 29: 56-62, 1973.

SCHOOL PHOBIA:

Coolidge, J. C., et al.: A ten-year follow-up study of sixty-six school phobic children. Am J Orthopsychia 34: 675-684, 1964.

Coolidge, J. C. and Brodie, R. D.: Observations of mothers of 49 school phobic children: evaluated in a 10-year follow-up study. J Am Acad Child Psychia 13: 275-285, 1974.

Kahn, J. H. and Nursten, J. P.: School refusal: a comprehensive view of school phobia and other failures of school attendance. Am J Orthopsychia 32: 707-718, 1962.

Miller, L. C. , et al. : Comparison of reciprocal inhibition, psychotherapy, and waiting list control for phobic children. J Abnorm Psychol 79: 269-279, 1972.

Schmitt, B. D. : School phobia - the great imitator: a pediatrician's viewpoint. Pediatrics 48: 433-441, 1971.

Waldfogel, S. , et al. : The development, meaning and management of school phobia. Am J Orthopsychia 27: 754-776, 1957.

SEXUAL ABUSE OF CHILDREN:
SEXUAL ASSAULT AND INCEST:

Bender, L. and Grugett, A. : A follow-up report on children who had atypical sexual experiences. Am J Orthopsychia 22: 825-837, 1952.

Giarretto, H. : Humanistic Treatment of Father-Daughter Incest. In: R. E. Helfer and C. H. Kempe (Eds.). Child Abuse and Neglect: The Family and the Community. Cambridge: Ballinger Publishing Co. , 1976, pp. 143-162.

Glaser, K. : Masked depression in children and adolescents. Am J Psychother 21: 565-574, 1967.

Jaffe, A. C. , et al. : Sexual abuse of children. Am J Dis Children 129: 689-692, 1975.

Kaufman, I. , et al. : The family constellation and overt incestuous relations between father and daughter. Am J Orthopsychia 24: 266-279, 1954.

Rosen, I. : The Pathology and Treatment of Sexual Deviation. London: Oxford University Press, 1964.

Sarles, R. M. Incest. Ped Clin N Am 22: 633-642, 1975.

Sloan, P. S. and Karpinsky, E. : Effects of incest upon the participants. Am J Orthopsychia 12: 666-673, 1952.

SEXUAL ABUSE OF CHILDREN:
INDECENT EXPOSURE AND INDECENT LIBERTIES:

Jaffe, A. C. , et al. : Sexual abuse of children. Am J Dis Children 129: 689-692, 1975.

SEXUAL IDENTITY PROBLEMS:
FEMININITY IN BOYS:

Green, R.: Sexual Identity Conflict in Children and Adults. New York: Basic Books, 1974.

Stoller, R. J. Male Childhood transexualism. J Am Acad Child Psychia 7: 193-209, 1968.

SLEEP DISORDERS: NIGHT TERRORS:

Fisher, C., et al.: A psychophysiological study of nightmares and night terrors. The suppression of stage 4 night terrors with diazepam. Arch Gen Psychia 28: 252-259, 1973.

Keith, P. R.: Night terrors - a review of the psychology, neurophysiology, and therapy. J Am Acad Child Psychia 14: 477-499, 1975.

SUICIDE AND ATTEMPTED SUICIDE:

Conger, J. J.: Adolescence and Youth: Psychological Development in a Changing World, 2nd Edition. New York: Harper and Row, 1977.

Macdonald, J. M.: Homicidal threats. Am J Psychia 124: 475-482, 1967.

Mattsson, A., et al.: Suicidal behavior as a child psychiatric emergency. Arch Gen Psychia 20: 100-109, 1969.

Morrison, G. C. and Collier, J. G.: Family treatment approaches to suicidal children and adolescents. J Am Acad Child Psychia 8: 140-153, 1969.

Shaffer, D.: Suicide in childhood and early adolescence. J Child Psychol Psychia 15: 275-291, 1974.

UNMARRIED PREGNANCY:

Aug, R. G. and Bright, T. P.: A study of wed and unwed motherhood in adolescents and young adults. J Am Acad Child Psychia 9: 577-594, 1970.

Kantner, J. and Zelnick, M. Contraception and pregnancy. Fam Plan Perspec 5: 21-35, 1973.

Konopka, G.: Young Girls: A Portrait of Adolescence. New York: Prentice Hall, 1976.

Meeks, J. E.: The Fragile Alliance: An Orientation to the Outpatient Psychotherapy of the Adolescent. Baltimore: Williams and Wilkins Co., 1971.

Miller, W. B. Sexual and contraceptive behavior in young unmarried women. Primary Care 3: 427-453, 1976.

Paul, E. W., et al.: Pregnancy, teenagers, and the law. Fam Plan Perspec 8: 16-21, 1976.

Semmens, J. P. and Lamers, W. M.: Teenage Pregnancy. Springfield, Ill.: Charles C Thomas, 1968.

Zelnick, M. and Kantner, J.: The resolution of first pregnancies. Fam Plan Perspec 6: 74-80, 1974.

THE VIOLENT OR AGGRESSIVE CHILD
OR ADOLESCENT:

Bandura, A. and Walters, R. H.: Adolescent Aggression. New York: Ronald Press, 1959.

Bender, L. Children and adolescents who have killed. Am J Psychia 116: 510-513, 1959.

Camp, B., et al.: Think aloud, a program for developing self-control in young aggressive boys. J Abnorm Child Psychol 5: 157-169, 1977.

Conger, J. J.: Adolescence and Youth. New York: Harper and Row, 1977.

Duncan, J. W. and Duncan, G. M.: Murder in the family: a study of some homicidal adolescents. Am J Psychia 127: 1498-1502, 1971.

Eron, L. D., et al.: How learning conditions in early childhood, including mass media, relate to aggression in late adolescence. Am J Orthopsychia 44: 412-423, 1974.

Freud, S. (1920): Beyond the Pleasure Principle. Standard Edition, Vol. 18. London: Hogarth Press, 1955.

Hartman, H. , et al.: Notes on the theory of aggression. Psychoanal Study Child 3-4: 9-36, 1949.

Hebert, F. B.: Psychiatric Emergencies. Paper presented at Denver Postgraduate Institute in Emergency Medicine, Denver, May, 1977.

Jenkins, R. L.: Classification of behavior problems of children. Am J Psychia 125: 1032-1039, 1969.

King, C. H.: The ego and the integration of violence in homicidal youth. Am J Orthopsychia 45: 134-145, 1975.

Lewis, J. A.: Violence and epilepsy. JAMA 232: 1165-1167, 1975.

Lorenz, K.: On Aggression. New York: Harcourt, Brace and World, 1966.

Macdonald, J. M. Homicidal threats. Am J Psychia 124: 475-482, 1967.

Rosen, H. and DiGiacomo, J. N.: The role of physical restraint in the treatment of psychiatric illness. J Clin Psychia 39: 228-232, 1978.

Tooley, K.: The small assassins: clinical notes on a subgroup of murderous children. J Am Acad Child Psychia 14: 306-318, 1975.

CHILD - ADOLESCENT PSYCHOPHARMACOLOGY

Abbott Laboratories, North Chicago, Illinois, 60064.

Campbell, M.: Treatment of Childhood and Adolescent Schizophrenia. In: J. M. Wiener (Ed.). Psychopharmacology in Childhood and Adolescence. New York: Basic Books, 1977, pp. 101-118.

Conners, C. K.: A teacher rating scale for use in drug studies with children. Am J Psychia 126: 884-888, 1969.

Conners, C. K.: Organic Therapies. In: A. M. Freedman, H. I. Kaplan and B. J. Sadock (Eds.). Comprehensive Textbook of Psychiatry 2nd Edition Baltimore: Williams and Wilkins Co., 1975, pp. 2240-2246.

Fieve, R.: Lithium (Antimanic) Therapy. In: A. M. Freedman, H. I. Kaplan and B. J. Sadock (Eds.). Comprehensive Textbook of Psychiatry 2nd Edition Baltimore: Williams and Wilkins Co., 1975, pp. 1982-1986.

Fish, B.: Drug use in psychiatric disorders of children. Am J Psychia, Feb. Supplement, 124: 31-36, 1968.

Frommer, E. A. Treatment of childhood depression with antidepressant drugs. Brit Med J 1: No. 5542: 729-732, 1967.

Hollister, L. E.: Clinical Use of Psychotherapeutic Drugs. Springfield, Ill.: Charles C Thomas, 1973.

Klein, D. F. and Davis, J. M. Diagnosis and Drug Treatment of Psychiatric Disorders. Baltimore: Williams and Wilkins Co., 1969.

Lehmann, H. E.: Pharmacotherapy of Schizophrenia. In: P. H. Hock and J. Zubin (Eds.). Psychopathology of Schizophrenia New York: Grune and Stratton, 1966, 388-411.

McAndrew, J. B. et al.: Effects of prolonged phenothiazine intake on psychotic and other hospitalized children. J Autism Child Schizo 2: 75-81, 1972.

Mann, H. B. and Greenspan, S. I. The identification and treatment of adult brain dysfunction. Am J Psychia 133: 1013-1017, 1976.

May, P. R.: Treatment of Schizophrenia. New York: Science House, 1968.

Prien, R. F. and Cole, J. O.: High dose chlorpromazine therapy in chronic schiophrenia. Arch Gen Psychia 18: 482-495, 1968.

Safer, D., et al.: Depression of growth in hyperactive children on stimulant drugs. New Eng J Med 287: 217-220, 1972.

Wiener, J. M.: Summary. In: J. M. Wiener (Ed.). Psychopharmacology in Childhood and Adolescence. New York: Basic Books, 1977, pp. 217-221.

INDEX

Haldol, 23, 146, 147, 148, 149, 150
Haldol, in violent children, 134
Hallucinations:
  hypnagogic, 115
  hypnopompic, 115
Hallucinogen intoxication, treatment, 22
Hallucinogens, in acute drug abuse, 12
Haloperidol, (see Haldol)
Hartmann, H., 128
Hebert, F. B., 54, 133
Helfer, R., 39
Heller's disease, 40
Herbert, M., 4
Heroin, 13
Hertzig, M., 46
High speed driving, 56
Hingtgen, J., 42
Hippocrates, 84
Hirsch, S., 57
Hoekstra, M., 9
Hoffmann, H., 78
Hollender, M., 57
Holter, J., 35
Homemakers, 109
Homicide, 129
Homicide and suicide, 134
Horowitz, H. A., 50, 54
Hospitalization:
  activities during, 94-95
  communication during, 94
  explanation of:
    to child, 93
    medications, 93
    procedures, 93
  follow-up treatment of, 96
  group meetings for, 95
  hypnosis in, 95
  psychotherapeutic treatment during, 96
  reactions to, 88-102
    appetite loss, 90
    child's, 90
    delirium, 91
    depression, 90-91

examination of parents in, 89-90
family equilibrium, effect on, 89
parents, 90
psychotic, 91
regression, 90
sleep disturbances, 90
treatment, 92-96
treatment, immediate, 92-96
use of play, 93
special treatment of, 95
visitations, 93-94
Huntington's chorea, 76
Hydroxyzine hydrochloride, 143
Hyperactive children, in adolescence, 141
Hyperactivity, 78-83
  caused by mental retardation, 80
  developmental, 79
  examination of child in, 81-82
  examination of parents in, 81-82
  fetal wastage, history of, 81
  "neurological", 80
  neurological examination in, 80
  parental management of, 81
  parents' history in, 81
  perinatal history in, 82
  psychogenic, 81
  "soft signs" in, 80
  treatment of:
    child psychotherapy, 82
    diary of events, 82
    educational, 82-83
    parent counseling, 82
    pharmacological, 83, 139-142
    role of teacher in, 82-83
    target behaviors, 82
    unproven, 83